WINNING
LIKE
YUVRAJ

Alpesh Patel is a published author, a consultant, an entrepreneur and a mentor to start-ups, with over twenty years of corporate experience.

Alpesh worked as a management consultant with the Big 4 accounting firms for fifteen years and advised corporates and governments on business strategy, technology, change management, mergers and reforms. As a consultant, he advised companies in the banking, insurance, micro-finance and power sectors. He worked on many greenfield ventures, including India's first payments bank, the country's first integrated steel plant and a telemedicine start-up that brought medical consultations to rural patients.

Alpesh is an engineer from the National Institute of Technology, Rourkela, and a management graduate from the S.P. Jain Institute of Management and Research (SPJIMR), Mumbai. He currently lives in Mumbai and manages a venture that focuses on leading technologies like artificial intelligence and robotic automation.

WINNING LIKE
YUVRAJ

THINK &
SUCCEED
LIKE
SINGH

ALPESH PATEL

RUPA

Published by
Rupa Publications India Pvt. Ltd 2018
7/16, Ansari Road, Daryaganj
New Delhi 110002

Sales centres:
Allahabad Bengaluru Chennai
Hyderabad Jaipur Kathmandu
Kolkata Mumbai

ISBN: 978-93-5333-289-1

First impression 2018

10 9 8 7 6 5 4 3 2 1

*Dedicated to the fans of Yuvraj Singh
for their continued love and support.*

Contents

Yuvraj Singh: The Survivor Prince of Cricket

In 1981, when Buckingham Palace announced the engagement of Prince Charles and Princess Diana, and later their fairy-tale wedding, India was gifted with a modern-day prince of its own. Yuvraj was born to Yograj and Shabnam Singh on 12 December. But like another prince, Siddhartha, he was to stay away from the public eye for a long time. But his entry into the public domain would grab the attention of several million people, not just in India but across the world.

Right from school, Yuvraj—or Yuvi, as he is fondly called—was inclined towards a life of sports and showed little interest in academics. He was always eager to be on the field and would head straight to the sports ground after school, getting back home only in time for dinner. Maybe it was that sports helped him push the limits of his body and mind, but Yuvi found himself engrossed in skating, football, tennis and cricket right from his early days.

However, it was his father Yograj Singh who persuaded

him to choose the world of professional cricket. An eminent personality in Punjab, Yograj was himself a former cricketer, who had played six one-day internationals (ODIs) and one test match for India as a right-arm fast bowler. Unfortunately, an injury ended his sports career and he found himself in the Punjabi film industry. He urged Yuvraj to focus on cricket, despite the latter being skilled at tennis and skating too. In fact, Yuvi had already won a gold medal in skating—one of his favourite games at the time—at the age of ten. He had even acted in a Punjabi film, *Mehndi Shagna Di,* in 1992, when he was just eleven. He could have continued to work in the film industry too, but he gave everything else up to be in cricket—and never, even for a day since then, has he thought of doing anything else. His life became cricket and cricket became his life. That is how the prince of Indian cricket—Yuvraj Singh—made his way into the collective consciousness of millions of Indians.

Yuvi's parents helped him throughout his cricketing career. Despite differences between them, they managed to shape a bright future for their son. Yograj was a strict disciplinarian, bordering on dictatorial at times, but despite this, Yuvraj benefited from his father's influence. Yograj was a skilled trainer and wanted his son to get what he couldn't—a long, successful career in cricket. Though this is every father's wish, to have his children follow in his professional footsteps, it does not always work out; but in this case, Yograj found in his son an equally—if not more—passionate cricketer. Yograj set up a strict training regime for his son and expected him to start performing right from an early age. He set up a cement wicket in his backyard, where he trained his son throughout the day. Lights were installed to help them practise even at night. Though he may have put Yuvraj through some unpleasant experiences, Yograj, through his experience and expertise, ensured that his son went on to become one of the country's leading cricketers.

However, legacy alone does not ensure success—as the sons of many famous cricketers have known—and despite Yuvraj's rigorous training and his father's support, he had to struggle before he could make it big in cricket. Many trainers with whom Yuvraj worked in his early days wrote him off. A few former cricketing giants also expressed doubt in his capabilities. But neither Yuvraj, nor his father gave up—and Yuvi climbed his way up the ladder of Indian cricket one step at a time.

Starting with domestic cricket at the age of thirteen, he represented Punjab for U-16 matches and then entered the state's U-19 team. In 1996–7 he made his debut in the first class with a match against Orissa (now Odisha) in the Ranji Trophy. In January 2000, Yuvi represented India in the U-19 World Cup and, by the end of the year, at the age of eighteen, he was made part of the ODI team for the 2000 ICC KnockOut Trophy. There was no looking back since then. He became part of India's test squad and, with his stellar performances, consolidated his position in India's ODI team. Later, after 2007, he sparkled in the Twenty20 (T20) and Indian Premier League (IPL) formats too.

During his upward journey spanning more than one and a half decades, Yuvraj achieved incredible highs and gave cricket fans some of the game's most memorable moments. But his career at the domestic level remained his backbone. Despite having to stay out of the team at times due to injury or loss of form, Yuvraj always made it back. Anyone who follows cricket will know how difficult it is to make a 'comeback' if one leaves the team even for a short period. But every time he lost his position in the team, Yuvraj's sheer grit and determination—apart from the support he enjoyed from the Board of Control for Cricket in India (BCCI), his family and his fans—brought him back. He would look into the problem, fix it, return to domestic cricket and give stellar performances every time. This made it difficult for the selection committee to ignore him for long, and Yuvraj remained a name to be reckoned with in the Indian cricket team for years.

A UNIQUELY ILLUSTRIOUS CAREER

Career statistics

Yuvraj's career statistics are indeed impressive. In first-class cricket, he played an overall 134 matches and amassed 8,866 runs, with an impressive highest score of 260. His batting average stands at 45.23—remarkable, to say the least—and in total, he has 26 hundreds and 36 fifties to his name.

His ODI career—packed with equally great performances and numbers—started with not just an impressive innings, but also a responsible one. Yuvraj is one of the very few cricketers to have had the privilege of getting a debut match during an ICC trophy tournament. It was the first quarter-final at the ICC KnockOut in Nairobi in 2000, and India, playing against Australia, had batted first. Unfortunately, none of the Indian batsmen managed to hit even a half-century, and the fate of the game rested on Yuvi's young shoulders. He made 84 runs off 80 balls, with a strike rate of 105. He hit 12 boundaries in that match, and India managed 265 for a loss of 9 wickets, eventually going on to win that match. Yuvraj's presence on the field was noticed by many that evening. From there on, he went on to represent India in several international matches, gaining the love, respect and support of fans worldwide.

Yuvraj's ODI career spans 304 matches and 8,701 runs, putting him among the top ten ODI run scorers in India. His highest in a match is 150. With a strike rate of 87.7, he emerged as one of India's most briskly scoring batsmen. That apart, he has a total of 14 centuries and 52 half-centuries to his name, along with 908 boundaries and 155 sixes—that is 4,562 runs in boundaries and sixes alone. That his runs scored in boundaries and sixes are more than half of his total ODI runs says a lot about his batting style. It was this flair for the game that saved India from many a humiliating defeat and helped him carve a niche for himself in the team. In a career spanning more than 17 years, Yuvraj has played in several batting positions, but in most matches, he has batted four or five down, where he has been a truly effective batsman. Of his overall 8,701 runs, about 6,500 were scored playing in that position. It is interesting to note here that the total number of runs scored by him at both the international and domestic levels is roughly the same.

Yuvraj is known not only for his prowess with the bat, but he has contributed noticeably in the bowling and fielding departments as well. In his 304 ODI matches, he has taken 111 wickets for India. Here's why this is a big deal—Yuvraj is one of the only three Indian players to have scored more than 8,000 runs in ODIs and taken more than a 100 wickets (the other two are Sourav Ganguly and Sachin Tendulkar). Yuvraj has bowled more than 5,000 balls for the team; his best is when he took five wickets after conceding just 31 runs. He also has two four-wicket hauls to his name.

Yuvraj has been an excellent fielder as well. He was one of the early players in the team to push the limits of conventional fielding. His lightning-fast reflexes have led captains to trust him with the most crucial positions on the field, something that many cricketers dread. To let a catch fall is to earn the wrath of several thousands of Indian cricket fans. But Yuvraj has steadfastly held these risky positions, confident that the ball will not pass through his hands at any point.

In his ODI career, he has taken 94 catches, of which his fans still remember the one in his debut tournament. The quarter-final against Australia in the ICC KnockOut was crucial to the team. Ian Harvey had been promoted to No. 3 to make some quick runs, and it looked like he would be a threat to India. Yuvraj was posted at cover. Harvey tried hitting Venkatesh Prasad for a lofted drive over cover, but Yuvraj flung himself through the air and took a catch that was not only visually impressive but also physically challenging. This iconic catch sent Harvey back that day, and India won the match, with Australia falling short by 20 runs.

But one of the most important moments in his career was in the 2016 IPL season, when Yuvraj was playing for the Sunrisers Hyderabad (SRH). When Royal Challengers Bangalore (RCB) and SRH took each other on for the trophy in the finals, the crowd was prepared for what one calls a T20 encounter. SRH won the toss and decided to bat first. They managed to set a target of 209. Yuvraj performed impressively, hitting 38 off just 23 balls, which included two sixes and four boundaries, and a massive strike rate of 165. When RCB came to bat, though, they were off to a good start. Chris Gayle held the crease for a long time, hitting a stunning 76 off 38 balls, with eight sixes and four boundaries. His strike rate was a whopping 200. But the game changed direction when Ben Cutting got his wicket and Barinder Sran got Captain Virat Kohli's. Players in their form were dismissed for nothing. A.B. de Villiers, Lokesh Rahul and Shane Watson were all sent back to the pavilion earlier than expected, and SRH eventually won with a tight eight runs.

Yuvraj's cricketing career has indeed been extraordinary. As an ODI batsman, he is among the top ten run scorers of India; he is among the top five Indian all-rounders of all time; and he is easily one of the best fielders India has had. But he is so much more than just his on-field statistics. And it's these aspects of Yuvraj Singh's personality and career that offer unique lessons on how to win like him—both in cricket and in life.

Title wins: his love for the big platform

No matter how great a cricketer's individual career record is, he will always crave big title wins, such as the World Cup. So imagine how special Yuvraj's career has been that he has won not one, not two, but three World Cups, and that, too, in three different formats. In 2000, it was the U-19 World Cup; in 2007, it was the T20 World Cup; and in 2011, it was the ICC World Cup. This is a feat no other Indian cricketer has achieved—not even Tendulkar, Ganguly or Rahul Dravid. Apart from the World Cups, Yuvraj has also been part of the Indian team that won the ICC Champions Trophy (jointly with Sri Lanka in 2002) and IPL in 2016.

It is not that Yuvi has just been lucky to be part of these winning teams. In all of these, he has played significant roles, as his Man of the Match/Series titles indicate. This brings us to the next aspect of his career that stands out.

Man of the Match/Series awards

Since the start of his career in 2000, Yuvraj has grabbed 27 Man of the Match (MoM) awards. That is an average of more than 1.6 awards a year! No wonder, then, that Yuvraj ranks at No. 14 in the list of cricketers with the most number of MoM awards in the history of world cricket. And it's not just in individual matches—Yuvi has sparkled in entire tournaments as well. In the 71 cricket series that Yuvraj has played, he has been chosen Man of the Series (MoS), seven times! That puts him among the top seven cricketers in the history of the game to gain this honour. Clearly, Yuvi is an 'impact' player, who makes his presence felt through his performance on the field. More importantly, he loves to deliver on big platforms, when the stakes are high. In the ICC World Cup that India won in 2011, Yuvi was adjudged the MoS. In the list of the top ten MoM award winners in World Cup tournaments, apart from Tendulkar, Yuvraj is the only Indian batsman with four MoM awards.

Yuvi's consistently top-class performance in big tournaments makes him unique among those who have similar—or even better—overall statistics in ODI cricket. For anyone who aims to be a lead contributor at the highest level, there are valuable lessons to be gained from Yuvi's success in big tournaments.

Overcoming challenges

The other fascinating aspect of Yuvraj's career is his comebacks.

Of course, over his 17-year-long career, Yuvraj, like any other player, has had phases where he has lost form or has had to sit out due to injuries. In 2006, he sustained a nagging knee injury, and in 2009, he fractured a finger in his right hand, which troubled him for a few seasons. Then, in 2010, when playing in Mirpur, Yuvraj had a ligament tear in his left wrist. His career hit a low in 2010, when, for the first time in ten years, he was dropped from the ODI team for the Asia Cup. But not one to take no for an answer, Yuvraj made a brilliant comeback in 2011, when he was chosen for the ICC World Cup. India not only won the tournament but Yuvraj was named the MoS. From getting dropped from the ODI team to being an anchor in the Indian team that won the World Cup is some comeback indeed!

But even as he celebrated this achievement, there was a sinister health problem brewing. Yuvraj hadn't given much thought to the coughing spells, sleepless nights and sudden pains that had ailed him throughout the 2011 World Cup tournament—but it was evident to many others, who had seen him spit blood on the field. It came as a shock not only to Yuvraj but to the entire world when Yuvi was diagnosed with cancer. His fans prayed fervently as he underwent treatment in the United States. The few photographs that were made available in the public domain during this time were widely circulated in the Indian media, and thousands of young men and women posted on social media, praying that their idol return to the field to take world cricket by storm again. The interviews that people gave after visiting him or the tweets they posted came as drizzles in a desert devoid of any hope or joy. But Yuvraj came back. As he always did. Through sheer grit and determination, and the support and love of his fans, Yuvraj started the second innings of his life.

The once-unbeatable cricketer started afresh and struggled all over again to regain lost ground. He worked to achieve the desired fitness level, while at the same time practising to hone his skills. And in September 2012, he made a grand re-entry into Indian cricket, when he played a T20 match against New Zealand. This was undoubtedly one of the bravest battles the generation witnessed, and Yuvraj's fight became a defining moment in his career, lifting him to the status of a man far bigger than the game.

But maintaining form wasn't easy. After his 2012 return to cricket, Yuvraj had a rather unimpressive record in 2013. Though he played T20 and IPL from 2014 to 2016, he did not secure a place in the Indian ODI team in this three-year period. This would ordinarily spell doom for a cricketer's ODI career, especially if he is in his late thirties, but Yuvraj, being the king of comebacks, did not give up. Yuvraj prepared relentlessly for his return to the ODIs—and then, in the 2016–17 Ranji Trophy, stunned India once again when he scored 672 runs for Punjab in just five matches. This included a double century and a ton—and became his ticket into the ODI team. By this time (2017), much in the Indian cricket scene was changing—M.S. Dhoni had resigned as captain of the Indian team and Virat Kohli had taken his place; India, too, had woken up to Yuvraj's return to the ODIs at the age of thirty-six. But allaying all his fans' fears, and surpassing all expectations, Yuvraj, in January 2017, scored his career best of 150 runs in an ODI against England in Cuttack. The world was dumbstruck and all naysayers were silenced. Had anyone ever seen such a comeback? How did Yuvi manage this? We shall learn in the subsequent chapters.

A compassionate star outside the cricket ground

As one can imagine, cancer changed Yuvraj's life. Those solitary moments spent during treatment perhaps made him realize the pain an illness can inflict on a person, and he developed the urge to inspire and help others who were braving similar fights. So Yuvraj started an NGO in 2012 called YouWeCan, to work towards raising awareness about cancer and helping needy patients financially. The organization reflects Yuvraj's conviction that early diagnosis and the right treatment can help people fight cancer better. The NGO website, at one point, stated, 'We at Yuvraj Singh Foundation believe in the dignity and potential of every life, through a self-aware, responsible and proactive approach towards a cancer-conscious society with an attitude to fight back in time.'

Yuvraj himself actively participates in the events of the NGO and can be seen engaging with children. People are delighted to see their hero as an embodiment of inspiration even outside the field, interacting with them and inspiring them to fight their battle against cancer. With YouWeCan, Yuvraj proved that one could excel and inspire even beyond the field and play a larger role in society. With this, he joined celebrities such as Shabana Azmi, Rahul Bose, Milind Soman, Nandita Das, Gul Panag, John Abraham, Nafisa Ali and Akshay Kumar, who have contributed to different causes at various points in their career. Speaking about inspiring millions, Yuvraj said, 'Earlier on in my career, it was more about cricket and now it is being more about inspiring people to come out of the adversity and create examples... Since my treatment, things have changed a lot for me.'[1]

In the phase post his cancer treatment, Yuvraj also engaged in various commercial enterprises to contribute to society and the country. This compassionate side also found expression in his business ventures—he wanted to help young entrepreneurs and their start-ups by funding their ventures. Talking about this idea, he said, 'I had been thinking about this for four-five years. There are a lot of young entrepreneurs with great, high-potential ideas and I plan to invest in these start-ups, to build their brands and companies.'[2] In 2015, he gave shape to his plan to invest crores of his own funds into start-ups and, over a period of three to five years, raise a few hundred crores from other sources towards his goal. It's not that cricketers have not been known to invest their money in some form of business, but investment into venture funds is not that common.

Yuvraj has tried to ensure that young Indians are able to contribute to the nation through backing from a personality like him. YouWeCan takes care of everything from brand-building and strategizing marketing campaigns to the monetization of business models. In the process, it has attracted a large number of entrepreneurs. Beauty service ventures and start-ups in the fields of logistics, healthcare, edtech, and online marketplace for chartering private jets are just a few examples in which YouWeCan's clients have gained immensely. This contribution to the nation's economy has earned Yuvraj even more respect among fellow Indians.

A star loved by millions

There are great performers in every field, but only a few acquire iconic status. Yuvraj is loved by millions because he is more than just a skilled cricketer—he is dedicated, hard-working, classy, compassionate and a master of comebacks, who has never given up chasing his dreams. The audience may not remember all his innings and all his big hits, but they will never forget how he revealed that the 'someone special' for whom he wanted to win the 2011 World Cup was none other than Tendulkar. His fans will never forget how he hit 6 sixes in a single over by Stuart Broad and how he made a comeback after defeating cancer. His fans will always remember the smiling face of a cricketer who always wore jersey No. 12 because his birthday is on 12/12 (12 December) and because he believes 12 is his lucky number.

It is no surprise that there have already been talks to showcase his life in a Bollywood biopic, so he can continue to inspire generations even after his time. Many directors, actors and producers have expressed their desire to be part of this; actors such as Abhishek Bachchan, Ranbir Kapoor and Emraan Hashmi have been reported to have shown an interest in playing Yuvraj on screen. Interestingly, Yuvraj had once said that he had Akshay Kumar in mind for the role. On a talk show, Yuvi had said, 'Well, I don't know who relates to me the best but as a Punjabi boy I think Akshay fits in that category.'[3]

In 2017, a US-based firm, Apex Entertainment, was reported to be planning to produce a documentary on Yuvraj's life. The president and co-founder of the firm, Mark Ciardi, had said, 'I have always believed in our company's philosophy of bringing aspirational stories from the world to you; characters who overcome adversity, stories that inspire minds... He [Yuvraj] is an inspiration to a billion Indians and cricket fans globally, the way he faced odds in his life and career, the way he survived cancer and the way he fought back to earn his place in the Indian team.'[4]

As fans await a film on his life, Yuvi continues to inspire thousands across India. Other than the love of his fans, Yuvraj has received various awards for his career. In 2012, the Government of India presented him with the Arjuna Award, a moment of great pride for not only Yuvraj and his family, but the entire cricketing world. It proved yet again that if one persevered, recognition was bound to follow. In 2014, Yuvraj was given India's fourth highest civilian award, the Padma Shri. Then, in 2017, a Gwalior-based university awarded him a degree in Philosophy Honoris Causa for his 'extraordinary sporting prowess and as a catalyst of change with great integrity and humility'.

CAN WE, TOO, WIN LIKE YUVRAJ?

Yuvi's life and career are in many ways exemplary. And during my research, these are some of the aspects of his life that I found worth learning from.

How to choose a passion

Just like in Yuvraj's case, when one is young, one is attracted to various activities, be it in sports, science or adventure. There are many role models as well. But to excel in any field, one needs to choose one passion and put everything else aside. Obviously, this choice is crucial. So how does one choose the right passion, the right career? Should one choose popular fields such as cricket and films, or should one take risks in relatively new or unknown fields? Should one live their own dream or should one allow parents to influence their choice?

Learning Tip
To excel in any field, choose
one passion and put everything else aside.

How to be a lead contributor in your field

From one hundred and thirty crore Indians, only fifteen boys are chosen to represent India in a cricket team. In a corporate career, too, as one grows, there are only a few roles in senior positions—and only one CEO in a company of, say, a thousand employees. Only those who can consistently contribute survive in the long run. So how does one keep shining in the team by playing match-winning innings, scoring centuries, grabbing wickets and taking the most catches in the field? How can one keep earning the tag of MoM year after year?

A never-say-die attitude

There will always be challenges in one's professional and personal life, often of the kind one has little control over. Yuvraj sustained injuries and was diagnosed with cancer when he was at the peak of his career. Such incidents can frustrate, even break people, and comebacks are not as easy as they sound. It is never a good feeling to be sitting at home with a plaster on the leg while watching others take your place in the team. But what helps stars like Yuvraj to rise even after they have fallen?

Being an all-rounder but focusing on one's strengths

If one is multiskilled, one is always urged to excel in more fields than one. Haven't we all seen those smart boys and girls in school and college who are everywhere—participating in quiz competitions, sports, adventures, dramatics and academics, all with the same gusto? But does participating in so many things at the same time help, especially at the start of one's career? When should one put a break on trying out too many things and choose stability in one field? Should one aim to be an all-rounder or focus on just a few skills? Yuvraj, too, had to face these challenges in life—be it in the choice of sport or in excelling at all formats of cricket, such as ODI, T20 and test.

Backing class with commitment

Sports stars such as Yuvraj, Diego Maradona and Roger Federer are gifted with style, grace and skill. They are classy, which has earned them a huge fan following. But to achieve greatness, class isn't enough; other factors such as commitment, a fighting spirit, confidence and ecosystem support are critical too. Yuvraj was always classy, but he backed this up with undeterred commitment. But how does one go about it?

Balancing commerce with compassion

We hone our capabilities and skills to achieve commercial success—that's how CEOs, film stars and sports stars harvest record earnings throughout their careers. Yuvraj earned record bidding in IPL in 2014, 2015 and 2016, but he wasn't just basking in the glory of contracts worth crores of rupees. He knew the importance of balancing compassion with commercial success. After all, when he was going through a bad phase in his own life, it was the care and love of his parents, coaches, doctors, friends, gurus and millions of fans that kept him going and gave him the courage to make a path-breaking comeback. After his treatment, Yuvi, too, reciprocated with compassion by opening an NGO for supporting cancer patients. The ability to win and give back compassion is what makes capable people true heroes and great brands. In the coming chapters, we will see how Yuvi succeeded in doing just that.

Learning Tip
Being classy is important, but back this
up with undeterred commitment.

Chasing His Passion

Didn't we all have a burning passion in our teens? While some wanted to pilot airplanes, others wanted to play for the Indian cricket team, while still others wanted to become the country's top cop. But how many of us actually pursued our passions? Not many. There are always hundreds of role models and dozens of thrilling ideas, but not too many are focused and determined enough to choose and chase just one dream. While there is no shame in not knowing what one wants to do even till late in life, latching on to a passion early has its own advantages. And that is what Yuvi did.

Like any other kid, Yuvi, too, had various interests, especially in sports. The naturally athletic Yuvi enjoyed football, tennis and cricket, but roller skating had a special place in his heart. While some would say that all young boys enjoy sports at that age, Yuvraj's aptitude was on a different level. He didn't just play for fun but gave his heart and soul into roller skating. No wonder, then, that even before he entered his teens, he achieved sporting glory, winning the national U-14 gold medal in roller skating.

It is a day that is etched into Yuvraj's memory—but for reasons he did not quite expect. That became one of the last occasions that Yuvraj was to ever set foot inside a skating rink again. As the tournament came to an end, Yuvi waited impatiently for his father to pick him up, unable to mask his excitement at having won gold. But what happened next changed the course of his life. Yograj looked away and threw Yuvi's medal out of the car, warning him, 'From now on, you will play cricket, not this girls' sport. If you don't play cricket, I will break your legs.'5

That was perhaps the evening cricket became a permanent fixture in Yuvraj's life, relegating everything else to second spot. In the years that followed, cricket became Yuvraj's only love, only passion. Thus, very early in life, he made a choice, even if it was determined by his father.

But why did Yograj treat his son's spectacular success in roller skating with such disdain? Perhaps the former cricketer had old scores to settle. Like all cricketers, Yograj had dreamt of making it big in cricket, but when he failed, he was well past his prime—and his world seemed to be crumbling. He now only had his son to resurrect it for him. His broken dreams of playing cricket could only be fulfilled by Yuvi.

So whether Yuvi liked it or not, his fate was sealed. From then on, he wasn't allowed to play any other sport but cricket. He was to train hard and make it to the Indian team, and make it big. All Yograj's bitterness was channelled into moulding his son into an ace cricketer.

Ironically, Yuvraj wasn't fond of cricket in the beginning. But slowly, he grew to love the game. A few years back, while he was being treated for cancer, he would constantly watch his innings on television, holding his bat. He found renewed passion in the game, and his love for cricket made him want to recover and return to the field. In those dark, lonely moments, cricket became his only light, his only purpose in life. That was how passionate he grew up to be about cricket.

But this single-minded focus and passion didn't happen overnight. Apart from sports, he also acted in films, like his father Yograj, who, after his career in cricket crashed, went on to become an established Punjabi actor, with films such as *Vichhora*, *Bhaag Milkha Bhaag* and *Jaat Punjabi Daa* to his credit. So, gradually, out of Yuvi's many interests, only one passion crystallized. Call it his father's choice or a classic work of fate, his life turned towards cricket. And he never looked back.

Managing early losses and training hard

Choosing a passion is only the first step. What comes next are the challenges—getting the right coaches, training hard to hone one's skills, aligning one's natural strengths with the right technique and handling early failures. So how did Yuvi do all this?

Interestingly, though Yuvi was always a good athlete, he wasn't superbly skilled at playing cricket from the beginning. He wasn't exactly a born 'master blaster', who could win India World Cups and become a prominent and inspirational cricketer from the get-go. Yograj put his son through intense training but also needed a good coach for him. However, several prominent cricketers of the time refused, as they did not see much promise in Yuvraj as a cricketer.

Yograj had got Yuvi admitted to Patiala's Yadavindra Public School. The Maharani Club cricket pitch, which was just a ten-minute walk away, was renowned as the training ground for former Indian cricketer and famous commentator Navjot Singh Sidhu. Yograj believed what his son needed was exposure, and requested Sidhu to train him. But when Yuvi got bowled on a full toss, Sidhu didn't feel encouraged. He watched for a while and then turned to Yograj, shaking his head. Sidhu told him blatantly that the boy was no good at cricket, and would never be.[6] Yograj stood silent for a while, absorbing the blow, but tapping into some hidden reserve, he let the feedback go unheeded and asked Yuvraj to pack his bags. He looked his son in the eye and said, 'Let's see how you *don't* become a cricketer now.'[7]

Passion is a strange concept. It makes you want to push back against the world's judgement, attempt the impossible and do what it says you cannot. And Yograj did just that, as if his life depended on it. In a way it did. So he got Yuvi back to Chandigarh. The beautiful garden that Yuvi's mother had made in their yard was turned into a 17-yard pitch, complete with floodlights. Even after dark, when the world prepared to go to bed, if one happened to walk past their house, one would see two figures in the yard outside—the bigger one hurling wet tennis balls (they hurt, don't they?) at the smaller one, who would be trying to save himself with a cricket bat. The young boy was allowed to spend less than half an hour with his friends every day. Apart from that, it was just training, and hard training, far from the relaxed cricket young boys play. It was work, and it was pain. But sometimes passion needs to be kindled and forcefully nurtured; it needs to be protected from the gusts of wind that threaten to blow it out, until it transforms into a raging fire. For Yuvraj, his father played that role.

For a good five years, Yuvi trained under his father at the DAV school, where the latter was a coach. Yuvi had to run in the morning and again in the evening at this ground. Yograj's training was relentless, and to top it all, with the practice pitch right in their backyard—literally—Yuvi could train any time of the day without even having to go to the ground. Yograj would throw wet tennis balls at his son, so that he could perfect his shots. He also took his son to the ground maintained by the Sports Authority of India (SAI), where, at the nets, he had fast bowlers throw bouncers to a helmetless Yuvi. The balls hit him on the back, neck, arms and legs. They must have made him cry out in painful frustration, filled him with anger; they may have even made him hate his father. But years later, this was the training that made him the Yuvraj Singh who could unflinchingly look Brett Lee in the eye as the fuming bowler sprinted towards him from the opposite crease, and smack the 140-kmph ball for a straight boundary. It was this training that made him fearless—he could let the ball hit him if it had to, let the pain run through his body. He had gotten used to it, but if it touched the bat, it would go for a six.

This harks back to one of Yuvi's practice sessions at the school. By now his commitment to cricket was evident to everyone. His attendance on the cricket field was higher than in class, and the way he played had started to give people a glimpse of the hitter he would become some day. It is said that Yuvi once hit so many sixes that the board on which the name of the school was written fell off the wall.

But there's another anecdote, this time involving none other than the great former cricketer, Bishan Singh Bedi. In the summer of 1993, when Yuvi was just twelve, his father had sent him to train under Bedi. The sweltering heat of north India was nothing less than torture for the boys on the training field. With sweat dripping down his face, and his jersey soaked, that was the first time Yuvi tried his hand at bowling. But after his first ball, Bishan Paaji told him he would never make a bowler of himself, and that he should never try. 'Go bat,' he had told him, and Yuvraj was dispatched to the other end of the pitch.

But the next summer, Bishan Paaji moved his camp to the small, sleepy town of Chail, tucked away in the mountains of Himachal Pradesh. Maybe it was the sparkling Himalayan sunshine, or maybe it was the beauty of the towering mountains, but that day, Yuvi scored his first hundred. Call it pride or boyish passion, or perhaps the hunger for more, but right after he scored that hundred, he went on to hit two more sixes. It was only after the second one that Bishan Paaji announced that if he hit another six, he would be declared OUT. He couldn't keep producing fresh cricket balls every time he dispatched one down the thousand-foot valley!

Yet, hunger kept Yuvraj going. He always wanted to do better. Better than everyone around him. And then move one step higher—and repeat. His hunger was insatiable. Of course, there were times when his mind revolted—he didn't want to train, he didn't want to work out, especially on chilly winter mornings when the temperature in Chandigarh would barely cross $1\,^{\circ}$C. Why couldn't he remain in his comfort zone for once, curled up in his warm blanket? But it is said that the comfort zone is a dangerous place; no growth ever happens there. And who would understand that better than Yograj?

One cold January morning, as his father came to wake him up, Yuvi continued to sleep. He listened with delight as his father's footsteps faded away in the distance. But the very next moment, he had a bucketful of ice-cold water emptied on him. There, shivering in his cold, soaked bed, Yuvi developed a kind of fear against the comfort zone, the very fear his father had hoped to instil in him.

But with every passing day, through his gruelling training sessions, he came to love the game. Though his father's unyielding discipline became a bit much at times, his growing love for the game led him to enjoy even those hard practice sessions. However, there came a time when he had to grow beyond his father's regime and train under other coaches in different conditions. The first such decision came in 1997, when he moved to Mumbai for training. One wonders how far he would have gone if he hadn't made that choice and continued to stay in Chandigarh. In Mumbai, he trained in Elf Vengsarkar Academy. Yograj had a close friend in Makarand Waingankar, who hosted Yuvraj in Mumbai during his training. It toughened up the young champ. Not only did he stay away from his father, but he also travelled long distances for training every day. He would have to travel miles just to get to the training ground. The oppressive humidity of the coastal city and the travel wore him down, it made him cry as he dragged himself to the field. He found himself complaining, but then he saw the other boys doing the same—young, aspiring cricketers fighting it out, battling to make a mark, but without the slightest hint of pain on their faces. And then he understood. And that day, he made a choice—to pursue his dream and not buckle under pain. A choice that would make him the man he grew up to be.

As a batsman, Yuvi was a powerful stroke player, who liked to lob the ball and send it flying high through the air. That was perhaps his natural style and testimony to his strength. But he was often advised to play close to the ground to avoid getting caught. But for Yuvraj, therein lay the fun! He played the ball close to the ground when his coach was around, but once he was gone, he would unleash his trademark stroke and hit the ball high up in the sky. Watching it soar lit up those eyes that harboured wild dreams of hitting the ball right out of the stadium while playing for India—dreams people would laugh at then, dreams so profound that one would think that the young boy was out of his mind. But then, that's the funny part about dreams—it is always the dreamer who gets to decide if they will become a reality. What could be termed delusions if unrealized, had the power to make the young boy a champion loved by the entire nation.

An incident that helped shape Yuvraj's on-field personality was when he was playing a Ranji practice match in Chandigarh. Yuvi smacked the ball up and high, just as he liked it. But as he was often warned, such shots came with risks: his shot had elevation but not enough distance, and caught out by the fielder, he walked back to the pavilion with a modest score of 39. When his father learnt how Yuvi had got himself out, shaking with anger, he told his wife to not let Yuvi enter the house that night. Shifting from one uncomfortable position to another, Yuvi spent a sleepless night on the back seat of their old Maruti car parked in the neighbouring sector. It was a never-ending night, but as the hours dragged by, he learnt an important lesson. He realized that instincts were good to ride on, but technique and control were equally important to play a long innings. The next morning, as the sun rose, he got out of the car a different man—a more responsible player who would control his natural instincts if required, a batsman the team could count on, a player who would spark hope in the hearts of millions even in the middle of a crumbling line-up, and one who would hear fans say that if Yuvraj was at the crease, India still stood a chance.

Yuvraj made his first-class debut for Punjab as an opener on a cold February morning in 1997 in Mohali, when he was just fifteen. The match, against Orissa, was the most important of his life until then. Debuting as a senior, the stakes were high, the pressure even higher. Even in the cold morning air, he could feel sweat beading his brow. And then the worst thing happened. He got out for a duck. That wasn't all: when it was time to field, he dropped a catch and then let the ball slip between his legs another time. He didn't have the courage to face his father. He didn't go home that night.

The next morning, tears of frustration stung his eyes when he read the newspaper headlines—Yuvraj Singh: India Gate, alluding to India Gate-like 'holes' in his fielding. The ball that had slipped between his legs had proved too costly. Quick as a flash, the haters surrounded him. The naysayers laughed. Like father, like son, they said—just like the father, the boy would never make it big. Imagine a career with such a horrendous debut. Wouldn't most of us lose hope? Give up? Go on to pursue easier goals? A different job? Yuvraj, too, could have opted for junior cricket, where the stakes were not as high, and where the odds were in his favour. But no. Yuvraj knew there was only one thing to do. He dusted himself down and started all over again. It wasn't easy. It took him two long years, but he kept working and sweating it out.

For the most part of the next three years that he spent trying to represent Punjab, he was made to sit out of the field. The seniors were often nasty, but Yuvraj swallowed his anger and bore it all with deep breaths and clenched fists. His patience, though, bore huge returns. In November 1999, on a turning wicket, he got his break. Playing against Haryana on that cold morning at the Nehru stadium in Gurgaon, he made a hundred. And suddenly, just like his first hundred in the Himalayan town of Chail, he felt like a thirteen-year-old all over again—light and carefree, soaring with the wind, soaring with the sixes.

That was an age before the mobile phone became ubiquitous, and every evening Yograj would call up on the landline in the dressing room and ask Yuvraj how he had played that day. The day Yuvi scored a hundred, he hovered around the phone like an excited kid, waiting for his father's call. The phone rang, but when Yuvi told him about his century, his father remained calm at the other end. Yograj asked him why it had been just a hundred—why not a double hundred? And just like that, Yuvraj's hunger grew.

Making his passion his career

It was Yuvi's hunger that led him to success. Yuvraj broke on to the professional cricket scene when he was just thirteen, in 1995, representing Punjab for the U-16 matches. Soon after, he made an entry into Punjab's U-19 team, where he shone by scoring 137 unbeaten runs against Himachal Pradesh. Then, in 1996-7 came the next milestone, when he played his debut first-class match against Orissa in the Ranji Trophy. But his first truly memorable game came in 1999 in the U-19 category at the Cooch Behar Trophy final, in which Punjab took on

Bihar. If Yuvi was the star of the Punjab team, guess who was leading Bihar? Dhoni. Dhoni scored a respectable 84 runs, but his team was all out for 357. When the Punjab team came to bat, Yuvraj alone hit 358 runs! Yes, he alone scored more than the Bihar team combined. As a result of his spectacular performance, he was able to make a laudable transition to international cricket.

In January 2000, sixteen teams participated in the third edition of the U-19 World Cup, which was being hosted by Sri Lanka. The tournament was to prove the announcement of Yuvraj's arrival on the international cricket scene. A player's performance in the U-19 World Cup is often the deciding factor in his selection for the national team. Harbhajan Singh, Mohammad Kaif, Virender Sehwag, Irfan Pathan, Suresh Raina, Rohit Sharma, Ravindra Jadeja and Virat Kohli have all in one way or the other risen from their U-19 international matches.

India had not won a U-19 World Cup for a long time, but the new millennium brought with it new hope. India, under the captaincy of Kaif, made fans swoon as they stayed unbeaten throughout the tournament, dominating in every aspect. In the semi-finals, they had a spectacular victory margin of 170 runs against Australia. In the finals, despite the Sri Lankans playing on home ground, India won by six wickets, sweeping away the cup. Guess who the hero of the Indian team was? Yuvraj Singh, who also won the Man of the Tournament award. He had played eight matches and scored 203 runs at an unheard-of strike rate of 103. But that wasn't all. He had also taken 12 important wickets. Kaif and Yuvraj had had a splendid partnership that they would go on to replicate in other formats of the game too.

That tournament, a star was born.

And Yuvraj Singh, the eighteen-year-old all-rounder from Punjab, was selected in the Indian squad for the 2000 ICC KnockOut Trophy. His first international match was an ODI against Kenya in the pre-quarter-final but, interestingly, he only got to bowl and not bat. He bowled four overs and conceded 16 runs. The next match against Australia, a quarter-final, was technically his first match as a batsman, and Yuvraj's performance in the very first innings earned him a list of admirers who would stay with him throughout his career. Imagine facing the world's best seamers—Glenn McGrath, Brett Lee and Jason Gillespie—in a debut match! Wouldn't that be intimidating? But Yuvraj played them all with unbelievable ease and went on to hit 84 runs off 80 balls. In his very first batting performance in an international match, he was given the MoM title.

With this, Yuvraj ensured that his place in the Indian cricket team was sealed, at least for the immediate seasons. This performance in 2000 was considered so iconic that many years later, on the occasion of Yuvraj's 300th ODI, Sachin Tendulkar would fondly remember this maiden knock. Tendulkar said, 'That [his debut] was a special innings by Yuvraj Singh. On that day, I remember it was overcast conditions and we decided to bat against Australia, and we went after their opening bowlers and got off to a good start and Yuvraj Singh took over... That was a big game as Australia dominated... They were miles ahead of everyone else. To beat Australia required a mega performance...'8 To hear Tendulkar say those words was one of Yuvraj's biggest recognitions before his 300th match.

It is said that when one works hard to get to a position they have long dreamt of, it helps not just the person but also others around him. Yuvraj's selection into the Indian cricket team can also be considered a similar example, thus turning the fortunes of not just Yuvraj himself and his family, but also that of the team, the nation and thousands of Indian cricket fans.

At the time of his 2000 debut, the Indian team was mired in controversy. India was fresh out of a match-fixing scandal and Mohammad Azharuddin, the former captain of the team and one of India's most talented batsmen, was banned from the sport for life. Ajay Sharma, Ajay Jadeja, Dr Ali Irani (the physiotherapist) and Manoj Prabhakar were also banned for five years. Lakhs of Indian fans who had looked up to these players were left feeling deceived and heartbroken. It would take a miracle to win them back. It was in this backdrop of shame and disappointment that Yuvraj made his debut in the Indian team. He was a godsend. Spectators and critics alike were left in awe of his prodigious backlift and exaggerated follow-through, along with his left-hander's elegance, which made watching him a treat. His batting seemed to be a blend of the fierceness of Lance Klusener and the flair of Brian Lara.

Yuvraj continued to show promise through 2002 with some impactful knocks. A special one was his 121-run partnership with Kaif in the NatWest series final match in England, when India was struggling to chase 326 runs. This match is also remembered for a bare-chested Ganguly waving his shirt from the balcony of the Lord's cricket ground. By now the Indian team had started winning matches abroad and Yuvraj had grown to play an important role in India's rise in the home-away series. Yuvi had now cemented his place in the team as a key middle-order batsman who could also bowl and field well.

After a mixed World Cup of 2003, where Yuvraj scored two half-centuries, India toured Bangladesh. Here Yuvraj hit his first century in the international arena—102 off just 85 balls, and remained unbeaten till the end of the game. Right after this tournament, the Yorkshire County Cricket Club, having witnessed his performance, selected him for their team. This feat had been achieved only by Tendulkar so far.

Over the coming years, Yuvi increasingly began to play a pivotal role in the team and demonstrated the art of successfully chasing high scores. In 2007, the introduction of a shorter form of cricket—T20—turned out to be perfect for Yuvraj's tendency to smash boundaries and sixes. His performance in the first T20 World Cup in 2007 proved that the format unleashed his passion and spurred him on to achieve incredible scores. In the Super8 stage of that tournament, in a match against England, Yuvraj left spectators spellbound by hitting six sixes in a single over by Stuart Broad and scored an unbelievably fast 50 in just 12 deliveries. Then, in the semi-final against Australia, Yuvraj, now in his element, scored a blistering 70 runs off just 30 deliveries. That evening, Brett Lee was hit for sixes, Stuart Clark was thrashed for boundaries and Andrew Symonds was treated like an amateur by Yuvraj. India went on to celebrate this new format of cricket by winning the World Cup and Yuvraj showed the world just how big he could score.

The launch of the IPL in 2008 brought with it the offer of captaincy for Yuvraj. However, although his matches weren't exemplary, he continued to perform well in the ODIs when playing for India. But then, in 2010, Yuvraj saw a lean patch and a loss of form. Many believed his chances of playing in the 2011 World Cup for India were diminishing. Fortunately for him, and for India, he was included in the squad—and Yuvraj went on to give a performance that everyone would remember with both bat and ball. In spite of being in poor form just before the World Cup, and suffering from the yet-undetected cancer, the 2011 World Cup proved to be the peak of Yuvi's career. Only his burning passion for the game could have pushed him to excel even in those circumstances. Indeed, performance comes easy when you are in good form, but it's excruciating when the odds are not in your favour.

Once Yuvraj's cancer was detected, he had to stop playing cricket, but he never once thought of quitting. After his successful treatment, a 'what next?' never crossed his mind. He would go back—to his passion, his game, the park, the bat, the dressing room and the fans who were waiting for him. So he picked up where he had left off and started training again. He played in the IPL seasons from 2013 through 2016 and went back to domestic cricket to prove his worth—again. His comeback to ODI cricket in 2017 was met with thundering applause from his fans. Surely, when Yuvraj looks back at his career now, he can proudly say, 'I had a passion, and I followed it.'

However, after his fight with cancer, Yuvraj started leaning towards another passion, apart from cricket. He decided to help those battling cancer. And for this, he set up his NGO, YouWeCan, for helping cancer patients, and then launched YWC Ventures, which focused on nurturing projects in the healthcare and the wellness space. And thus, Yuvraj the individual performer transformed into a leader with a social mission.

Choosing life's passions

Yes, if we want to succeed like Yuvraj, we need to steadfastly chase our passion. But, as we have discussed before, how do we *choose* that one passion? It's not easy. While growing up, we have various personalities we want to emulate; to add to that, our parents have their own plans for our future. And many times, their dreams may not coincide with ours. In the case of Yuvraj, he initially wanted to take up roller skating and tennis, but his father urged him to take up cricket and Yuvraj relented, albeit reluctantly. But soon, their visions coincided and Yuvi started enjoying the game. The advantage of taking the advice of parents is that one can benefit from their experience in making practical and safer choices. However, the disadvantage could be that parents can be restricted by their own backgrounds and biases, sometimes ignorant of their children's hidden potentials and the new opportunities the world offers.

The perfect choice, then, lies in the zone where the three elements—one's passion, one's abilities and market opportunities—meet. That is when one can enjoy a career that is both fulfilling and rewarding.

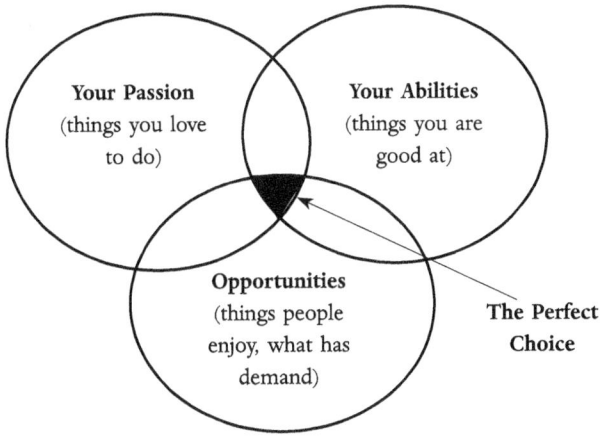

People who are happiest with their professions say, 'I am happy that my job requires me to do what I love. And I am lucky that I also get paid for it!' Yuvi made a successful career in cricket not only because cricket was his passion, but also because he had, or developed, the necessary skills for it; and the sport, being a popular one, offered him enough opportunity to flourish.

The often neglected element when choosing one's career is the innate desire in people to be admired and needed by society. It is human nature that we not only like to pursue what we love, but also feel appreciated for what we do. That does not mean that we should only choose fields such as cricket, films or music that are mainstream and already liked by the masses. We could also take up new fields (from an Indian perspective), such as sand art, adventure sports or athletics, and carve a niche for ourselves by creating something exceptional and world-class, thereby opening up new fields of excellence in the country.

But no matter what the goal, remember the golden rule—always chase your passion. The ultimate aim should be to become known for what you do by excelling at whichever passion you are pursuing. Just as Ustad Bismillah Khan is known for the shehnai, and Ustad Zakir Hussain for the tabla, Yuvraj Singh is known for being a cricketer his team can bank on.

So how quickly should one decide on one's passion? To find the right one, it is often a good idea to try one's hands at several things before settling for one and giving it one's best. This enables one to separate one's genuine passion from short-term fascinations and allows him/her to check if they have the required skills to excel in that field. There are instances where cricketers have been involved in other professions before switching to cricket wholeheartedly. Dhoni, for instance, played football before shifting to cricket. He worked as a train ticket examiner, more commonly known as the TTE, but dared to pursue cricket, and is now one of India's greatest cricketers. Ian Chappell, apart from being a celebrated cricketer, was also a successful baseball player. A.B. de Villiers played sports such as golf, rugby, hockey and tennis, and, in some, even played at the national level, but ultimately chose cricket as his passion. Mitchell Johnson, who is today known as an aggressive bowler, used to work as a truck driver transporting plumbing material in Australia. But in his spare time, he sharpened his bowling skills. Yuvraj, too, as we know, had other areas of interest before he switched to cricket with single-minded dedication. All in all, it is perfectly okay to initially not know what you want to do or dabble in various things before you zero in on a profession. But once you find your calling, you should work passionately towards excelling in it, leaving no stone unturned in being the best version of yourself in that field. That is what makes a real champion.

Learning Tip

Once you find your calling, you should work
passionately towards excelling in it.

Doing justice to your passion

Choosing a passion is only the first step, but how does one stay true to it? How does one keep achieving higher levels of excellence, the way Yuvraj did? And is this especially more challenging if one chooses a less popular field? Harsha Bhogale, an IIM graduate who could have easily taken up a corporate career but instead pursued the 'alternate career' of a cricket commentator, famously said that people focus on the 'alternate' part but forget the 'career' part of their passion. Choosing to do something different is exciting, but making a successful career out of it is indeed difficult.

But the toughest part is being able to sustain one's interest in it and maintain quality and focus. As Yuvraj's career highlights, succeeding in one's passion requires:

▸ Hard work
▸ The will to fight against adversity
▸ The ability to improve one's skills and overcome competition
▸ The temperament to enjoy what one does

During the 2011 World Cup, no one knew Yuvraj had cancer. Though people had seen him spitting out blood or vomiting during matches, they were only thought to be symptoms of stress, fatigue and strain, and nothing more. Yuvraj, too, went about it as if nothing had happened: he took sleeping pills for rest before big games, he tolerated unbearable pain both before and during matches, only so he could give the game his best shot. And he did. The pain, the blood-spitting and the vomiting were all unpublicized and known to very few. It was only later that it was discovered that Yuvraj had played with a cancerous growth in his lung. Doesn't this count as the ultimate sacrifice for the nation? When he played despite the pain, Yuvraj became a classic example of what it meant to love the game with his life—in his case, literally so. That year India won the World Cup but Yuvraj won hearts.

As one pursues one's passion, one needs to be sure to find joy in the journey. As the years pass, and passion becomes career, the excitement can dwindle, but one needs to keep one's interest in it alive. To do this, one needs to drive oneself to achieve newer milestones. The anticipation and excitement of living one's childhood dream is what keeps one going in one's career, like in the case of Yuvraj. Of all the matches he grew up watching, the India-Pakistan ones caught his attention the most. He dreamt of one day facing Wasim Akram on the pitch.

Learning Tip

As one pursues one's passion,
one needs to be sure to find joy in the journey.

And that day did come.

It is 1 March 2003, the day of the ICC World Cup match between India and Pakistan at the Centurion, and Yuvraj finds himself in the middle of a massive cricket ground packed with wildly cheering spectators. Standing on the crisp pitch, with its dazzling floodlights and the electric, almost deafening, atmosphere, he sees the man in green far down the ground hurtling towards him. It is Wasim Akram. As the seconds tick by, the speck grows bigger and more furious. Yuvraj feels his heart pounding against his chest, his heartbeat matching the rapidly advancing footsteps. He sees passion, focus and fury in his opponent's eyes. Around him, he can hear bits of commentary, like snippets from far away. 'Yuvraj Singh at the crease. Looking confident. Looking strong. Final ball of the match. Six runs to win. Will he make it for India? It's Wasim Akram to Yuvraj

Singh.' And then an eerie silence. An intense vacuum. All that is audible to him is the blood throbbing wildly in his ears. He looks down at the crease one last time. At his bat. At his blue jersey. The Ashok Chakra on his chest. The word 'India' in the middle. He takes a deep breath. The thousands in the stands hold their breath. The billion the world over, eyes glued to television screens, clutch their seats. Yuvraj looks up. He sees the white ball flying towards him. Fresh from the cannon. Closer. Closer. He swings his bat. The white ball cracks against its centre. That sweet sound. And the ball goes high up in the air. So high that he has to strain against the blinding floodlights to see where it goes. His heart jumps to his throat. He shuts his eyes. Moments tick by. In perfect silence. And then an earth-shattering roar. The crowd erupts into wild celebration. He is dazed. The speakers are blaring. At the other end of the pitch, the umpire slowly raises his hands. Not one, both. It is a six. India has won the match. Only then does Yuvraj come back to his senses, realizing that his childhood dream has indeed come true.

But there had been no butterflies in his tummy, like he had expected. It all felt perfectly normal—perhaps because he had trained for it with all his heart. That is perhaps how one feels when one has worked hard to get to one's goal. When years of effort have gone into something, when one is finally in the situation, there are no butterflies. Yuvraj said that Akram spoke to him after the match that day and congratulated him on the way he had played. Passion driven by diligence had made Yuvi's dream come true.

When one truly lives one's passion, as Yuvraj did, it becomes a purpose. And in bad times, that purpose becomes a reason to keep going: it became a reason for Yuvraj to live and get back to his life after cancer. As he lay on his bed in Indianapolis in the US, undergoing cancer treatment, he focused on cricket to take his mind off the pain. When dark thoughts and doubts plagued him, he sought peace and confidence in watching recordings of his knocks from past matches. It perhaps gave him a purpose in life all over again. He dreamt of returning to cricket and making it bigger than before. Rewatching those matches made him want to fight and live on. And when he reminisced about how he had pulled off those innings, which on hindsight seemed miraculous, it made him realize that he could, in fact, win this match against cancer too.

Man of the Match: Being the Lead Contributor

The inclusion of Yuvraj in the 2011 World Cup team was a gamble. His performance the previous year had probably been the worst in his career. His ODI average in 2010 was just 31.7 runs per innings, compared to the 45.9, 38.8 and 39.1 in 2007, 2008 and 2009, respectively. He was recuperating from injuries, and he was arguably not at his fittest. However, the selectors' gamble paid off, and Yuvraj more than proved his worth in the tournament, playing many innings crucial to India's victory. He was named the MoM in four matches, a feat achieved only by two others players in the past—Aravinda de Silva in 1996 and Lance Klusener in 1999. In the final against Sri Lanka, when the last shot, a six, was hit by Dhoni to chase out a winning total of 275 runs, Yuvraj was standing unbeaten at the other end of the crease. Such was Yuvi's presence and contribution to the tournament that he was adjudged the MoS as well. It was an acknowledgement of his contribution to the rare feat of India becoming the first country to win the World Cup on home ground.

On hindsight, Yuvraj's inclusion was the right decision, not because he was named the MoM or the MoS, but because he loved to excel on big platforms and flourished in challenging situations, often turning the tide of a match with his unshakeable grit and resolve. No wonder, then, that he has the enviable record of being the lead contributor in three of India's World Cup wins.

In every field, captains want heroes on their teams, especially in tough situations—lead contributors who often go on to win accolades at the highest levels. On the battlefield, the Gorkhas are among the fiercest fighters in the world. At the workplace, teams that have the best combination of skills and attitude are the most coveted. In the army, lead contributors win gallantry awards, while in the corporate world they are bestowed with the Employee of the Year medals (or the FIVE Ratings). In cricket, the equivalent is the MoM award.

Yuvi: A true impact player

The most noticeable aspect of Yuvraj's cricketing career is the number of MoM and MoS awards he has won. Indeed, he has repeatedly been the lead contributor in the Indian team for years. Or, as they say, he has been an 'impact player' in crucial matches.

Since the start of his career in 2000, in less than 17 years, he has grabbed 27 MoM awards. That is an average of more than 1.6 awards a year. Right from when he started playing for India in the international arena, until 2011, when India won the World Cup, there has not been a single year that Yuvraj has not got the MoM award. In all these eleven years, he has performed consistently as the lead contributor to India's victory. It is this consistency and reliability that has made all captains look forward to working with him.

Of his 27 MoM awards, six alone can be attributed to Yuvraj's matches against England. Yuvraj has consistently achieved milestones while playing against this one country, which include the six sixes in an over against Stuart Broad. Perhaps when Yuvraj was giving it back to Andrew Flintoff after a verbal face-off at the ICC T20 Cricket World Cup in 2007, he was also settling scores between the two countries.

All his MoM awards have come at crucial stages in the matches. In these matches, Yuvraj scored 13 tons and in eight, came close to scoring one. But not always has the environment been conducive to scoring runs. In cricket, the home advantage is crucial—the players are used to the pitch, the turn of the ball and the climatic conditions. Then there are the fans cheering for the home team. But the real test for a player is performing abroad, in conditions that may be uncomfortable to one's game. The pitch is different, the player doesn't know the rough and tricky patches, and there is a hostile crowd constantly booing the team. Indian batsmen generally struggle while batting abroad, especially in conditions when the ball swings a lot. But that was not the case for Yuvraj. Of the 27 MoM awards he has won, 13 have been won in matches played on foreign soil. The unyielding practice sessions with his father in the backyard, the long hours spent sweating it out on the pitch even as boys his age stayed comfortably indoors, and days keeping his cool against a hostile crowd that didn't think he would ever make it as a cricketer toughened him up to excel in any environment. This quality, which has many fans in awe of him even today, is one of the key factors that define a 'lead contributor'. Captains have time and again relied on Yuvraj to perform when the rest of the team has fallen apart. He has always seized the challenge and never backed out of a tough game. Yuvraj, through his consistent performances and incredible skill, has underlined the importance of being confident even outside one's comfort zone.

Yuvraj ranks fourteenth in the list of international players with the most number of MoM awards. Others on the list include stalwarts such as Tendulkar, Ganguly, Viv Richards, Ricky Ponting, Sanath Jayasuriya and Adam Gilchrist. Of the top twenty MoM award winners in international cricket, there are only four Indians—Tendulkar, Ganguly, Kohli and Yuvraj. And in the list of top ten MoM award winners in World Cup tournaments, apart from Tendulkar, Yuvraj is the only Indian batsman with four awards to his name. It is for this reason that Yuvraj has received nothing but praise from Indian cricket legends.

But Yuvraj has performed not only in single matches but in entire tournaments. Of the 71 series he has played for India, he has been chosen as the MoS seven times. This achievement has placed him among the top seven cricketers in the history of the game to have received this honour. Here again, he shares the privilege with his idol, Tendulkar. But what makes him rise even above Tendulkar in this case is the fact that he achieved this feat playing a fewer number of series than him. Interestingly, he won his MoS awards while playing against formidable teams. Two came while playing against South Africa (2005 and 2007), two more against Pakistan (2006 and 2007), one against England (2006) and another against Sri Lanka (2009). The last was in the 2011 ICC World Cup. Three of these awards were won in tournaments played outside India, again proving that he could excel in adverse conditions and opposite tough opponents.

The introduction of T20 cricket was followed by the IPL. It came not only as an incentive to cricketers but also as a yardstick of their own skills. IPL saw league owners select and reject players purely on the basis of performance, with little space for sentimentalism or favouritism. Yuvraj shone here too. In 2014, he was bought for a mammoth ₹14 crore by RCB. In this season, he made his T20 career-best score, a stunning 83 off just 38 balls. He also became the first all-rounder to register 50 or more wickets, and also capture four wickets in the same IPL season twice. He was rewarded for his performance by being bought in the next IPL season (2015) for a whopping ₹16 crore. All teams and league owners had by then realized that Yuvraj was one player worth bidding for, even if it meant shelling out huge sums of money. Everybody wanted Yuvraj in their team, making his bidding session one of the longest in that IPL season. Preity Zinta, Rahul Dravid, V.V.S. Laxman, Vijay Mallya and others at the auction were seen with tense expressions on their faces, trying to figure out a way to get Yuvraj on their side. It was a rather tough fight among Kings XI Punjab, RCB and Delhi Daredevils. The first to give up was Kings XI Punjab, and it was left to the Challengers and the Daredevils to fight it out. But Delhi had no second thoughts about bidding and it seemed that right from the outset, it had decided that it wanted Yuvraj on its team, come what may. It was RCB that found it difficult to decide. It could neither shell out so much money, nor let go of a player like Yuvraj. After a few minutes of intense discussion, RCB decided to let go, and Yuvraj, as rightly anticipated, went to Delhi. The Daredevils' captain, J.P. Duminy, realized Yuvraj's potential early on, as did the fans and owners of the team. Duminy was heard saying, 'I have no doubt that Yuvraj will win games on his own.'[9] The intensity of the bidding for Yuvraj speaks volumes about his winning calibre and perceived capabilities as a cricketer.

However, Yuvraj's on-field skills have not been recognized only in MoM and MoS awards, and IPL biddings. He was given a Porsche 911 by the vice president of the BCCI for his stellar performance in the 2007 T20 World Cup, Audi India presented him with a Q5 for his all-round performance in the 2011 World Cup, and in 2012, the Indian government honoured him with the Arjuna Award right after his comeback from cancer. In 2014, he was awarded the Padma Shri, India's fourth-highest civilian award, alongside three other sports stars—he was the only cricketer among them. The same year, he was given the Most Inspiring Sportsperson of the Year Award by the Federation of Indian Chambers of Commerce and Industry (FICCI).

So what makes Yuvraj a true MoM? If one had to pinpoint four qualities, these would be the ones that make him a distinctly big contributor in his teams:

- ▸ He loves the big platform.
- ▸ He performs under pressure.
- ▸ He contributes to the game even in pain.
- ▸ He is a team player.

Loving the big stage

There have been many instances when Yuvraj has not been in top shape for the game, but put in a big-platform tournament, such as ICC matches, he has instantly pulled himself up. The man simply cannot pass up an opportunity to rock on the big stage; one would think he even enjoys dealing with the pressures that come with it. Even as a boy, Yuvraj was hungry to get better. He always focused his energies on being the best in whatever he did, be it batting, bowling or fielding.

Of his seven MoS awards, the most important was arguably the one he got for the 2011 World Cup. This series was unforgettable for Indians for a number of reasons. Right from the time India was selected to host the World Cup, India had to put up a tough fight. In spite of cricket being akin to religion in the country, the Indian cricket team had won the World Cup only once before—in 1983, with a completely different set of players. It had been almost three decades since. It had managed to be a runner-up in the 2003 tournament, apart from reaching the semi-finals twice before—in 1987 and 1996. The drought was painful. It was high time that Team India won the cup for the nation.

What made the situation worse was that India's batting maestro, Tendulkar, was expected to retire after that year's World Cup. It would be a pity if, despite having so many records to his name, the man had no World Cup in his trophy cabinet. A tacit pressure started to build up on the Indian team to win, if only for the man considered the god of cricket by the world over. It was a question of pride for the Dhoni-led Indian team. It wanted to give Tendulkar the best World Cup farewell it could. Yuvraj, too, who had grown up watching Tendulkar play, wanted desperately to bring home the cup, more for Tendulkar than for himself. In fact, he had a picture of Tendulkar stuck inside his World Cup tournament kit, alongside his own. He looked at the picture every time he opened his bag to remind himself who he was doing it for. The entire team in 2011 was eager to lift the cup for the sake of one man.

The heat set in as the World Cup began. Yuvraj played with great proficiency and reliability. Against Ireland, he scored a half-century and grabbed five wickets, a feat not many have achieved in their careers. But Yuvraj's most important innings came in the quarter-final against Australia at Ahmedabad. He scored 57 important runs to help India chase the Australian total of 260 and make it to the semi-finals. It was the first time since 1992 that Australia had been knocked out before the finals. When India subsequently made it to the finals against Sri Lanka after beating Pakistan, it was the first time in history that two Asian countries were part of the World Cup final. But the stakes were even higher—never before in the history of cricket had a host nation won a World Cup playing on home ground. With the final match slated to be played in Mumbai, tensions ran high, as the home-ground advantage can easily turn into a disadvantage if things don't go well for the host country. The entire nation was watching, and a defeat would not only be ignominious but demoralizing for the team. In the nail-biting final, Yuvraj rose to the occasion with bat and ball, and watched gleefully from the other end of the pitch as Dhoni scored the winning runs. India became the first host country in the history of cricket to win the World Cup on its home ground. Fans went crazy, the streets felt like a carnival was under way, and people, not just in Mumbai, but in even the smallest town and hamlet in the country, went delirious with joy. It was a sight unlike any other. And if there was any man that night to whom the team owed the cup, it was Yuvraj. That day he became the first all-rounder in the world to score 300-plus runs and take 15 wickets in a single tournament. What a feat! He was rightly adjudged the 2011 World Cup Player of the Tournament. He scored a total 362 runs that tournament, with an average of over 90, including four half-centuries and one century. Out of the eight innings he played, he remained unbeaten on four occasions. The man for whom the team had won the cup, Tendulkar, was lifted on the team members' shoulders that night, and the happiness on Yuvraj's face was unlike any anyone had ever seen. Yuvraj had done it for the country and for the Little Master.

However, this wasn't the only World Cup of which Yuvraj was an integral part. In the 2000 U-19 World Cup, alongside Kaif, he had put up a tremendous show. His 58 off 28 balls against Australia in the semi-final remains unforgettable. He emerged as the star performer in the tournament, scoring a total of 203 runs, at a strike rate of 103; he also took 12 wickets at an average of 11.5. Yuvraj had learnt to be an all-rounder right from 2000.

He had also been part of the Indian team that won the 2007 T20 World Cup. His knock against Australia, where he scored 70 off just 30 balls, with an astonishing strike rate of 233, and the one against England, where he scored 58 off just 16 balls, with a strike rate of 362.5, are performances that stand out in cricket history even today. The latter holds the record of being the fastest fifty in an international T20 game—and it still stands unbroken.

Performing under pressure

They say when the going gets tough, the tough get going.

Almost anyone who has played advanced professional cricket can perform when the odds are in their favour, the stakes are not too high and victory is in sight. But what happens when the runs are not pouring in, the batsmen are struggling, the line-up is falling apart and the air is heavy with apprehension? That is when the team needs someone like Yuvraj, who can keep his cool and squeeze out victory from the jaws of defeat. These are the innings that matter the most. There is a thrill in rising to the occasion and winning one for the team, and for millions of fans. That is Yuvraj—always living on the edge. Every time he is asked about his favourite matches, he recollects games in which he had to play under pressure.

An interviewer once asked him how he managed to thrive under such intense pressure and he replied that such situations always brought out the best in him: he simply focused on what the team needed him to do and played his own game. And he always gave his 110 per cent to it.

Several of Yuvraj's innings stand out when we try to recollect his best games. For instance, the 2002 NatWest series finale, which became one of the defining moments of Yuvraj's career. Imagine a score of 326 to be chased down against the formidable England in its own den, Lord's. England obviously had an edge over India—a pitch they were accustomed to and an audience ready to fuel them with their enthusiasm. The Indian wickets began to fall, and the line-up crumbled under pressure. India was struggling at 146/5 at the end of 24 overs, when Kaif joined Yuvraj at the crease. Indian fans had already lost hope, but Yuvraj and Kaif created magic that day on the field and saved India from a humiliating defeat. Ball after ball they remained at the crease, and together scored 121 runs to steal the game from

England, before Yuvraj was dismissed for 69 off 63 balls. From a losing proposition, India went on to win that match by two wickets. And that wouldn't have been possible without Yuvraj. The look on Captain Sourav Ganguly's face said it all—he was ecstatic. If you were at Lord's that evening, or glued to the television set like millions of fans worldwide, you would have caught sight of Ganguly on the balcony taking off his jersey and waving it over his head in sheer delight. Consistent contributors like Yuvraj (and in this series Kaif) are indispensable if teams are to emerge as winners.

Another of those memorable instances was when India played against England in 2008. The England team toured India in November and December 2008, and played two test matches and five ODIs. During that time, the country was rocked by the Mumbai terror attacks, which left Indians grieving and the world appalled. Owing to the attacks, a few matches had to be cancelled to ensure the safety of the players. But even amid that tragedy, the Indian team came down heavily on the English side with a thumping series win. It brought cheer to a broken nation. Yuvraj, as always, was a big factor in the massive 5–0 ODI series victory. He won the Player of the Match award twice in that series. He scored consecutive centuries in Rajkot and Indore. He was superb, not just with the bat, but also with the ball. In the second ODI, he impressed everyone with a ten-over spell, grabbing four wickets and giving away just 28 runs. He turned out to be a lead contributor in that match too.

But in retrospect, what mattered more was the partnership he had with Tendulkar in the first test of the same England tour. Any Indian batsman would yearn to play such an important role in the team's victory, working alongside Tendulkar. England had won the toss and decided to bat first. The Indian team had managed to get them all out for 316. Yuvraj sent James Anderson back to the dressing room with an impressive catch. He had earned a wicket too. But the Indian batting side failed to perform, as they were bundled out for a shameful 241. India, facing a humiliating defeat, had to undo the damage in the second innings. England set a difficult target of 387, before confidently declaring. It was the final day of the test. Though Gautam Gambhir and Virender Sehwag looked promising, with an impressive start, they were sent back on 66 and 83, respectively. Dravid and Laxman, who were supposed to take over, also failed. They were sent back with single-digit scores. It was now up to Tendulkar and Yuvraj to save the day for the Indian team. And together they put up an impressive partnership of 163 runs. India won, and at the end of the match, Tendulkar and Yuvraj both remained at the crease unbeaten, at 103 and 85, respectively. This was the fifth highest test run chase overall and the highest in India. It is precisely in such tough situations that Yuvraj shines, not only for the game he plays but also for bailing out his team.

The list of Yuvi's memorable innings, in fact, begins right from the early period of his career. For instance, in the U-19 World Cup, the world saw one of the first examples of what Yuvraj was capable of. Australia had always been a formidable side—it didn't matter if it was the senior team or the U-19 team. In the semi-final match, India won the toss and decided to bat first. India put up a decent score of 284 in fifty overs. Yuvraj effortlessly scored 58 runs off just 25 balls, including five fours and five sixes. He was the only Indian batsman in that innings to have sent the ball over the boundary. He also had the best strike rate in the entire game. Where a few of the other batsmen hardly touched a strike rate of 100, Yuvraj boasted an impressive strike rate of 232. Australia was later reduced to 114 all out. Yuvraj also fielded brilliantly, taking two elegant catches. It's no wonder, then, that he caught the eye of many that day.

Playing a mature game, taking the pressure off his team and adding runs to the board mattered the most to Yuvraj, as is evident from the second quarter-final of the 2011 World Cup in the jam-packed Motera stadium of Ahmedabad, where India was playing against Australia. This time, too, luck seemed to favour the Aussies. India lost the toss and had to bat second. The Australians looked unstoppable and Indian skipper Dhoni had to try out multiple options to keep the Australians in check. He experimented with the ball, even letting Kohli and Tendulkar bowl. Yuvraj shared a third of the wicket toll with the other bowlers Ravichandran Ashwin and Zaheer Khan, both of whom had two wickets each. With 260/6, Australia stood a good chance of winning. On the Indian side, Sehwag and Kohli lost their wickets without much contribution, while Gambhir and Tendulkar both managed half-centuries. While one after the other the Indian batsmen walked down to the pavilion, Yuvraj stood steadfast on the crease and pitched in to compensate for the falling wickets. Later, along with Suresh Raina, he was able to lead India to victory with an elegant 57. He had hit the most number of boundaries in that game. For having ensured a berth for India in the semi-finals, he was rightly awarded the MoM award, the fourth time in that World Cup tournament. He said, 'I don't know about hitting any purple patch, but the pressure today, playing Australia, it was something else... When Dhoni got out, I knew we still had Raina to come, and thought if we added 40 odd runs it would be good... I have gone through a tough year, but coming into the World Cup, getting that 50 against England, it was good, 260 was a good score, Ponting batted outstandingly but we chased well.'[10]

His recognition of Ponting was a sign of the respect he had for good performance on the field, be it on any side. It is because of players such as Yuvi that the idea of cricket being a gentleman's sport has been retained. Ponting, keeping up the same spirit, reciprocated the gesture at the end of the game, when he praised Yuvraj for his performance as well.

No captain can deny Yuvraj's contribution to his team's victory, and the fact that he has, in many cases, been indispensable to the team is recognized by players, captains, coaches, selection committees, experts and the audience alike.

Even in 2017, despite everything, Yuvraj remained a lead contributor in the team. It was an India-Pakistan match—and like all matches between the strained neighbours, it was crucial to fans. It was 4 June and India lost the toss to Pakistan in the fourth match of Group B in the ICC Champions Trophy. Rain created havoc, but the game went on with periodical breaks. India had to bat first and delivered an impressive game. Rohit Sharma with 91, Shikhar Dhawan with 68 and Kohli with 81 managed to earn some early runs for the team. When it was Yuvraj's turn, he scored 53 runs in just 32 balls, with a strike rate of 166. With 8 fours, he was the player with the most number of boundaries in this match too. This tremendous knock came in handy to set a total of 319 for the Pakistani team. But rain interrupted the match, and the target was reduced to 289, which had to be attained in 41 overs. But India managed to destroy the Pakistani team at just 164 in less than 34 overs.

Despite there being other batsmen who had scored more runs, the Player of the Match award went to Yuvraj for his stellar performance. What really counts is how many runs a batsman adds when conditions aren't favourable and runs are most required—and Yuvraj was that saviour to the Indian team that day.

Contributing even in pain

Handling mental pressure in a game is one thing, but imagine playing with a body wracked by physical pain. Cricket has seen many instances in which players have been unable to perform due to pain or injury. In these circumstances, even though the player has the will and the skill, his body refuses to cooperate. But in India, two notable examples come to mind, where the players bent the body to their will to deliver ace performances on the field. The first is Anil Kumble in May 2002, when India, touring West Indies, was playing its fourth test. While batting at No. 7 in this match, Kumble was hit on the jaw by Mervyn Dillon. He spat out blood, but continued to bat for another twenty minutes. Nobody realized he had a broken jaw until it was examined later. India finally declared at 513 for 9. And when it was time to bowl, instead of choosing to sit the rest of the match out, Kumble had the Indian physiotherapist bandage his broken jaw at the boundary line, and then walked right back on to the field. He even sent Brian Lara back to the pavilion that day. This immense display of grit, passion and courage evoked new-found respect in the hearts of his fans. Kumble would later fly to Bangalore (now Bengaluru) the next day for surgery, but when asked why he had decided to risk so much and get back on the ground, he casually replied that he didn't want to sit around. Viv Richards, one of the greatest cricketers to have ever played the game, was nothing but praise for Kumble that day, noting that he had never seen such levels of commitment and courage before.

Yuvraj's was a similar case. In 2008, during the England tour of India, in the first match at Rajkot, India had to bat first after England won the toss. India got off to a good start, with Gambhir scoring 51 and Sehwag 85. Later, Raina pitched in with 43 off 77 balls. And then came Yuvraj's turn. To the world it seemed like any other innings he played, but only he knew he was playing with a muscle pull in the back. He could have given up, and nobody would have blamed him, but he played on through the pain and the agony—he clenched his fists and grimaced his way to a spectacular 138 off 78 balls. And what's more, he got the highest number of boundaries in that game too. With 16 fours and 6 sixes, he got a hundred off boundaries and sixes alone. The Indians performed adequately well with the ball and buried the English for 229 in just 38 overs. Yuvraj went on to be given the MoM award again. The English captain Kevin Pietersen said, 'At the end of the day when you stand up and watch an innings like that of Yuvraj…you just have to say "well played guys"… They played superb cricket…'[11]

Yuvraj himself was delighted to receive the award that day. And it was only after receiving it did he mention the muscle pull. This instantly made the world see him in a different light. We can't even walk around with a pulled back muscle, imagine playing an entire match with one, and also scoring a century— that, too, without complaining!

One of the biggest shocks to the cricketing world came

when news of Yuvraj's cancer broke. What truly makes him a hero in the eyes of the world is that he played the entire World Cup tournament with a tumour in his body. Often during matches he would run out of breath, gasping for air between two runs on the field. He would have intense coughing fits and would be seen spitting out blood. Some nights, it would be impossible for him to sleep, and yet, without letting the world know, he would take sleeping pills to get the required rest before a big game. Despite the pain and the sleeplessness, he would be up every morning to cheerfully be part of the game again. But in the end, with cancer still gnawing at his lung, he played a crucial role in India's victory in the World Cup and was awarded the Man of the Tournament trophy as well. When asked much later about it, he said, 'Yes, I was not doing well, I was coughing blood. It had started even on the South Africa tour before the World Cup. But I had to put the country first.'[12]

Each match was an internal war for him, but he pushed his body to the limit and tested its strength and resilience. This, apart from the immense pressure that playing for India at the international World Cup level brought. It is for this quality in Yuvraj that Indians hold him so dear. He could have pulled out of the tournament citing health reasons, and there would not be a single person in the entire nation who would have held it against him. But Yuvraj was not made of that stuff. He sacrificed his own well-being for the sake of the millions of Indians who were pinning their hopes on him, eagerly waiting to see India win the World Cup. What can you say about a man who doesn't even blink twice before deciding to make such a sacrifice?

Being a selfless contributor, always

Yuvi, over his career, has not only proved to be a lead contributor in the team but also a man who can be trusted with making the right choices on the field. And for that, he was appointed the vice captain of the team on several occasions. In 2009, during the T20 World Cup, when Sehwag was injured, Yuvraj was the first choice for the role of vice captain. However, though his fans were overjoyed, it seemed strange that he wasn't offered captaincy of Team India. However, Yuvraj himself didn't let it bother him much. His aim was to ensure the team's victory—be it as a captain, a vice captain or a player. And that's another thing about Yuvraj—he has never let such matters affect his game or his relationship with his captains. And when it comes to this attribute, he shares the stage with his idol and inspiration, Tendulkar. Yuvraj has played many an important knock under the captaincy of players who have once been his juniors, without the slightest grudge. It has never deterred him from giving a match his best. What has always mattered to him the most is the team's victory.

Learning Tip

Don't let ego get in the way of performance.

And one of the players he has shared a great rapport with is Dhoni. To the shock of many of Yuvraj's fans, in 2007, Dhoni was given the Indian team's captaincy, despite Yuvraj being senior. However, Yuvraj went on to become a crucial part of the team, working with his captain to ensure many an important victory for India. Dhoni, too, on his part, had played with Yuvraj long enough to know his strengths and worked on those to ensure Yuvraj could perform his best.

In 2009, Yuvraj was replaced by Kumar Sangakkara as the captain of Kings XI Punjab. There were allegations that Yuvraj's not-so-impressive performance was because he had been denied the role of captain. To this, Yuvraj said, 'When people said, I didn't perform because Sangakkara was made captain…it is a serious allegation—as serious as match-fixing. It was not acceptable and it was very hurtful… I was actually okay with playing under Sangakkara too. I am playing under Dhoni too.'[13]

Not being captain has never stopped him from carrying out his responsibilities as a senior member of the team, be it while playing against strong teams or helping the captain's on-field assessment of a situation. Many reporters at various points have asked him about his relationship with his captains on and off the field, and he has gracefully answered them on every occasion.

A reporter had once asked him, 'Even if you're not captain of the side, as you become a senior player in the team—and as people like Rahul Dravid, Sachin Tendulkar and Sourav Ganguly ease out of the game—you have a leadership role to play, don't you?' And Yuvraj had responded firmly, 'Of course. Being the vice captain of the team, I have to take as much pressure off Dhoni as I can. Being the vice captain, you see a lot of things on the field. You have to try and help the captain as much as you can and lead by example on the field. Small things like getting a run-out or taking a catch makes the other boys try and lift their standards. So yes, I do have an important role, even if I'm not captain.'[14]

Such words not only lift the morale of the entire team but

illustrate the level of maturity Yuvraj has when dealing with the game. That is what makes Yuvraj the lead contributor in the Indian cricket team.

But being a lead contributor doesn't come easy, whether in a sport, in a college competition or in one's professional life. Delivering at the highest level in pressure situations, such as, say, national-level competitions or mega-pitch presentations to big clients, requires not only the ability to handle pressure well, but also the aptitude for performing on big platforms. To emerge as a lead contributor at the highest level, one needs to have the maturity to accept different roles in a team without expecting to always be a leader or a captain. And to sustain the role of the highest contributor over a long period, one needs to learn to overcome adversities such as physical pain or emotional setbacks, and stay focused on contributing to the job at hand.

Learning Tip

One needs to have the maturity to accept different roles in a team without expecting to always be a leader or a captain.

King of Comebacks: A Never-Say-Die Attitude

Everyone has rough phases in their career. But our performance is dependent not just on our abilities and skills, but also on other circumstances that can overpower us. Sociopolitical conditions, health, family issues and rough competition are some of the things that are beyond our control most of the time. It is in times such as these that our confidence, willpower and ability to fight back are put to the test. Many of us give up at such junctures because we feel helpless, but what separates the ordinary from the extraordinary is the latter's ability to see these rough patches through.

Throughout history, there have been luminaries who have overcome crippling challenges with their never-say-die attitude. Abraham Lincoln lost elections more than eight times, lost more than one job and failed at numerous business attempts; to top that, he had a nervous breakdown. But if Lincoln gave up in these times, blaming the conditions around him, he wouldn't be remembered today. The story of *Harry Potter* author

J.K. Rowling is also familiar. She lost her mother at an early age, had a broken marriage, was unemployed and depressed, and was trying to raise a child on her own. After five long years of hard work, she approached publishers to get the first *Harry Potter* novel published. But she was rejected by twelve major publishing houses. It was much later that her manuscript was accepted for a meagre advance—and look at where she is today.

We have similar stories in cricket too. In 1999, Tendulkar lost his father just days before the World Cup match against Kenya, but he fought this emotional breakdown with a fabulous 140 that kept the Indian team afloat in the tournament. Kohli's case is poignant too. He was 40 not out in a Ranji Trophy match when news of his father's death reached him that evening. To everyone's surprise, he walked into the ground the next day and hit an impressive 90 to save Delhi from a follow-on.

Yuvraj, however, tops the list of those with a never-say-die attitude.

Interruptions in Yuvi's career

Yuvraj's career has been riddled with setbacks and challenges. To begin with, his early training with his father was brutal, to say the least. Though Yograj had good intentions, and can indeed be credited with shaping Yuvraj's determination to pursue cricket with single-minded focus, his rigorous discipline and strict training regime could have broken any boy. That Yuvraj not only withstood that kind of pressure, but turned it into a decisive driving force to do better is testimony to his greatness as a sportsperson and an individual. To add to this, he wasn't initially a great player—he was rejected by experts and written off by many due to his early bad innings. But that just pushed him to excel at the game. Didn't we say he liked to take on big challenges and emerge a winner? Anyone who would have known Yuvi in his early days would have noticed this attitude in him.

From his debut in international cricket in 2000 until 2007, Yuvraj had a fairly smooth run—his game improved, he added record after record to his name and his stature in the Indian team rose. It was only after 2007 that major challenges started cropping up. Still a young player at twenty-six, he sustained serious injuries in the next two years, but continued to give great performances in the IPL and T20 games, and no one challenged his position in the team. But things changed in 2010. His match statistics deteriorated and criticism started mounting. For the first time in a decade, he was dropped from the team for Asia Cup that year. Rightly or wrongly, he was accused of partying too much and drifting from the game. But soon after those criticisms, Yuvraj being Yuvraj, proved all critics wrong and gave the performance of a lifetime in the 2011 World Cup, in which he emerged as the MoS. But then came the worst setback of his life—the detection of a malignant cancer in his lung. Yuvraj took his first long break from the game in 2011–12 for treatment, but made a comeback in September 2012. But due to non-performance, he was out of the game from mid-2014 until early 2016, when he made a brief return to cricket. He was out again for about a year and then returned in January 2017.

What a challenge-filled career Yuvraj has had! A stressful introduction to the game in childhood, injuries at the peak of his career, criticism for a lack of focus, and then a battle with cancer. But through all of this, there has been one consistent aspect—his comebacks.

Bouncing back

Yuvraj hit his first lean patch in early 2005. In the first six months, he had played in eight matches but averaged a poor 17 runs per innings. Coach Greg Chappell came down heavily on him and media criticism was rife. Yuvraj had to bounce back. And he did. In August of the same year, in a match against West Indies in Colombo, when India was reeling at 51 for 3 (Ganguly was retired hurt), Yuvraj walked in and blasted 110 off 114 balls to lead India to victory. On reaching his century, he roared in triumph and gesticulated at the Indian dressing room. The tiger was back in killing form, with that performance marking the beginning of a stunning turnaround. Between November 2005 and May 2006, he hit 3 hundreds and 7 fifties in just twenty-two matches, averaging 62. This was the first instance where Yuvraj showed how stunningly he could bounce back from poor performance.

But his 2005 lean patch behind him, there came a series of injuries. In October 2006, Yuvraj sustained his first major injury, which caused a temporary interruption in his career. He was playing for India in the ICC tournament and a day before the match against Australia, he injured his left knee while playing kho-kho during the nets and had to sit out the rest of the tournament. It was a serious injury and though he initially tried to fix it with acupuncture, surgery was the only way out. He had suffered an anterior cruciate ligament (ACL) injury, which usually affects athletes in sports that demand extreme footwork, such as football and basketball. But for a cricketer to get this injury was a sign of the extreme effort that he put into training sessions and matches. Despite surgery being suggested by experts, Yuvraj tried his best to use various non-invasive methods so he could carry on playing. 'Operations aren't for me,' Yuvraj would say. He knew that surgery wasn't a magical quick-fix; rehabilitation would take long, which meant that he would have to miss at least five months of international cricket. He was having a great run and hence unwilling to take a break.

For the next tour of South Africa, Yuvraj was provisionally included in the team. The BCCI released a special statement clarifying that Yuvraj had been advised specific exercises and asked to use crutches to take some weight off the injured knee. The cricket board's medical consultant, Dr Anant Joshi, was to reassess the condition of his knee in two weeks, based on which the BCCI would decide on the next course of action.

Moving around in crutches is one of the most demotivating things for a sportsperson, but Yuvraj bore the mental agony in silence and bounced back in a few months. In January 2007, he was back in the team. In the third game after his return, he scored a magnificent 95 off just 83 balls against Sri Lanka and led India to a decisive victory. He was India's lead scorer, with 3 sixes and 11 fours, and had built an unbroken 145-run fourth-wicket partnership with Ganguly. The 2007 World Cup was just around the corner, and though Yuvraj was just back from a serious injury, he proved that he was in form and ready to be selected for the World Cup squad.

Though that World Cup didn't go too well for India, Yuvraj's performance proved that he had left the days of his injury behind. India unexpectedly lost an early match to an inexperienced Bangladesh team, which bundled the Indian side for a meagre 191 runs. Of this, Ganguly contributed 66 and Yuvraj 47, with three boundaries and a six. In the next match, against Bermuda, India came down heavily, thanks to the strong criticism the team had received for losing against Bangladesh earlier. India put up an impressive 413 with the loss of just five wickets. Ganguly and Sehwag scored 89 and 114, respectively; and Yuvraj, in just 41 deliveries, scored 83 runs. He hit 7 sixes in his innings and, like on so many other occasions, ended up hitting the most number of sixes in that game.

Unfortunately, India made an early exit from that World Cup, but Yuvi managed to make a good contribution with both bat and ball.

But soon after that World Cup, he injured his knee again—and this time it was worse. He got a combination of physiotherapy, osteopathy—which uses massage and bone manipulation—reflexology and other alternate methods, thanks to cricketer-turned-doctor Dr Jatin Chaudhary, whom Yuvraj called his 'miracle doctor'. The treatment was so successful that he recommended Dr Chaudhary to both Tendulkar and Sania Mirza for their injuries.

From 2007 to 2009, Yuvraj kept playing for India, with some discomfort from his knee injuries recurring from time to time. However, his career was largely uninterrupted. Towards the end of 2009, though, he faced a series of new injuries. In September that year, during a practice session in Johannesburg, Yuvraj fractured a finger on his right hand. This was a major setback and he was unable to play for India for six weeks, and eventually missed the Champions Trophy.

In December 2009, the finger injury continued to nag and

he missed the first two matches in the five-match Sri Lanka ODI series. When he played the third match, his injury aggravated, rendering him unfit to play the rest of the series. The new year didn't bring him any good news either. In January 2010, while playing the second test against Bangladesh in Mirpur, Yuvraj had a ligament tear in his left wrist. Coach Gary Kirsten announced, 'He has a torn cartilage on this wrist... Yuvraj will be struggling to make it for the first test against South Africa. He will be out for a while. But he will stay till the game ends.'[15] For Yuvraj, this came as a great loss. At an age when a batsman is supposed to be at his peak, Yuvraj was being constantly troubled by one injury after another.

In May 2010, Yuvraj played in the ICC World T20, but continued to struggle. India was knocked out in the Super8 stage by Sri Lanka. Yuvraj scored just 74 runs in five matches and stood at mid-wicket, usually reserved for mediocre fielders. He was now being criticized for his lack of fitness. He was dropped from the ODI squad for the Asia Cup, to be played in June. This came as an unpleasant shock to him and his fans. Further, since he was dropped less than a year before the 2011 World Cup, it raised uncomfortable questions about Yuvraj's form and whether he would be good enough for the World Cup. And even if he was, would he be free of injury? People waited anxiously to see where Yuvraj was headed.

Then, in August of the same year, India played the Triangular series with New Zealand and Sri Lanka. Yuvraj was included, but had nothing crucial to offer. In the same month, he got dengue and missed a few matches. Pressure was mounting and he had to perform to keep himself afloat.

Between the end of 2009 and October 2010, Yuvraj went

through one of the worst patches in his career, all thanks to injuries. He broke his fingers thrice, had a cartilage tear in his wrist, was troubled by his recurring knee injury and suffered a series of neck sprains.

In an interview, when he was asked how he looked back on that period, he was honest enough to confess that he wasn't in good form. 'Well, it has been full of injuries; my form wasn't great. I have struggled a lot throughout. But the year has made me strong mentally, because it was a tough year to go by. I would say the worst in my ten years of playing career,'[16] he said. Injuries apart, Yuvraj had also developed the image of someone who partied too much and wasn't as serious as a senior member of the team should be. To add to this, he was always in the middle of some kind of gossip or the other. He had to battle all of this to stage a comeback. When asked how he felt, he said, 'The back-to-back injuries left me emotionally and physically drained, and because of those injuries, I never got time to settle back into a rhythm.'[17]

Just when Yuvraj was seen as losing his grip on the game and his position in the team, he made the biggest comeback of his career. In September–October 2010, Yuvraj went for a three-week stint at the National Cricket Academy in Bangalore, equipped with the latest infrastructure for the training and rehabilitation of cricketers. From there, he went back to playing domestic cricket to try and get good match practice. In October, he went to play the Irani Cup, in which Rest of India was playing Mumbai in Jaipur. On the fourth day of the cup, he hit a crucial double century to come back in style. His knock raised the target his team set to a massive 782 for Mumbai. It had been more than twelve years since Mumbai had had to chase such an outlandish score. Yuvi was back after a year full of injuries and a dismal dry run without any international century. It finally looked like his 'toughest year' was coming to an end, and he was clearly ecstatic. At the end of that day, he said, 'I wanted to be back in form after a long layoff due to injuries. I am happy I did it... I was trying to play on the merit of the ball. The pitch was nice and the ball was coming nicely at the bat.'18 Yuvi had earned back his place in the Indian squad.

That October, in a match against Australia at Vizag, Yuvraj scored 58 runs. This was his first half-century in international cricket after a gap of ten months. Right after that, in November, India played against New Zealand. In the first ODI, Yuvraj hit 42 runs, with seven boundaries, and managed to grab 3 wickets, conceding only 43 runs. This was yet another day of all-round performance by Yuvraj. Three matches later, in the fifth ODI, he managed to get 2 wickets in 2 overs, giving away just 5 runs. He also managed to score 42 runs as a batsman. He sustained this form in 2011, as India toured South Africa. In the second ODI, he managed to get 53 runs off 74 balls, with four boundaries, and in the fourth ODI got India three wickets.

Yuvi was out of that disastrous patch, but he wasn't yet where he used to be. So when he was selected for the 2011 World Cup, the decision was much criticised. His disastrous run during 2010 was still fresh in people's minds. Many believed that he didn't deserve to be in the World Cup team and that the role should have been given to someone younger and fitter. But in the World Cup, people saw a completely different Yuvraj Singh. The effort he had put into improving his game was visible to everyone.

In the tournament, he hit 4 half-centuries and 1 century.

He hit 362 runs in just nine matches, at a staggering average of 90.5 runs per match, and also picked up 15 wickets. He became the fourth cricketer and the second Indian (since Kapil Dev) to achieve the double of 300 runs and 10 wickets in the same World Cup tournament. He was deservedly given the MoM award in four matches and also adjudged the Player of the Tournament.

He had not only made a comeback, but also scaled new heights. His perseverance and tendency to push his limits while practising at the nets had paid off. The Yuvraj who was so far known as the match winner, the charismatic player and the hard hitter was now also given the tag of the 'king of comebacks'.

But fate threw Yuvraj a new challenge—the most cruel so far—when he was diagnosed with cancer after the 2011 World Cup win. Before the group match against West Indies, he began vomiting blood and wasn't able to eat much, as he was throwing up most of what he was eating. Even on the day of the match, he felt dizzy. It is unusual for umpires to be involved in what is happening to players on the field unless reported, but Simon Taufel asked him that day if he wanted to leave the ground, given his condition. Yuvraj responded by saying, 'You can take me to the hospital if I fall or collapse, [but] until then, I am staying.'[19] The match had to be halted several times during the innings, as he threw up between overs, but that day he scored his highest in the tournament—113 runs in India's overall 268. Apart from this, he took two crucial wickets and sealed India's chances in the game, and was awarded the MoM. One can only wonder what would have happened if Yuvraj had taken up Taufel's offer to withdraw from the game. But his determination and perseverance not only saw him through the game but also helped him emerge as a crucial player.

After India's World Cup win, Yuvraj underwent a scan of the chest cavity. This revealed a tumour, but refusing to believe he had cancer—as that would mean he would have to leave cricket for good, or at least for a long time—he continued to play. It was only in January 2012, when another scan revealed a tumour the size of a tennis ball near his chest, that he was forced to face the fact that the tumour was malignant—a germ cell cancer called a mediastinal seminoma, located between his heart and left lung—and that it was growing. It had by then become about 14 centimetres.

He couldn't avoid the issue any longer and had to quit cricket. That very month he flew to Indianapolis for treatment. After several tests, he underwent chemotherapy from February to March, also getting Ayurvedic treatment at the same time. He made good progress and was sent for rehabilitation in May.

As soon as he was discharged in 2012, he trained his eyes on the Indian squad that was to play the T20 World Cup. He had to go through immense struggle to regain his form and practise harder than ever before. He tweeted a picture of his bald head, saying, 'Finally the hair has gone! But #livstrong #Yuvstrong.'[20] His tweets revealed his deep yearning to be back on the Indian team. On one occasion he tweeted: 'I will fight and come back as a stronger man cause [sic] I have the prayers of my nation! Thank you to the media for their support and respecting my privacy. And of course every day I look forward to come back and wear my India jersey, my India cap and represent my country again. Jai hind.'[21]

Finally, the much-awaited day came. In less than a year of his cancer treatment, on 11 September 2012, Yuvi played in the

T20 game against New Zealand. His fans were delighted to see him back. When he walked into the field, the crowd roared his name and gave him a standing ovation. Irrespective of which team they were supporting, each one in the stadium respected the kind of struggle he had had to go through before making it back to the field. He had fought cancer, defeated it, trained hard and managed to impress the strict selection committee. If there was any feat worthy of recognition, it was this.

In that match, he scored 34 runs, with a boundary and two sixes. It was classic Yuvraj Singh for the crowd. He shared a good partnership of 42 runs with Dhoni. Unfortunately, India lost the game that evening by just 1 run. When called on to speak, he said, 'There are mixed emotions... We lost a game that we should have won, but for me personally it was a big emotional moment to get on the field. I had tears in my eyes when we were fielding, luckily the cameras did not catch it. I think I am timing the ball well and it can only get better from here.'[22] One could sense the feeling of achievement and confidence that Yuvraj felt.

His comeback was lauded by everyone. Dhoni said, 'It was good to see Yuvraj come back and score some runs. It was a big game for him. I personally feel that he gives us the right kind of balance we need. He is not someone who will bowl all four overs in a T20 game, but he is a variation that I can use, especially since we have to play with four specialist bowlers.'[23]

Before the game, Yuvraj had tweeted, saying, 'I guess this would be my biggest day after World Cup final. I'm really overwhelmed with the love and support of everyone who have send [sic] me wishes.'[24] He also wrote on his Twitter handle that day, 'Few hours to go till I wear my fav jersey[...] To my mom my friends my fans this wud not bin pos thnks for ur lov nd courage.'[25]

But unlike other comebacks, this wasn't only about him, his family and friends. It was about so many more people, across towns and cities in India. It was a personal message of motivation to every cancer patient from Yuvraj Singh that day, when he tweeted, '...[I]f yuvi can u can fight cancer and come back wher u belong! So shout youwecan today all those who u survivors and r goin to survive ... For the cancer society! See u on the field and I hope it On the field! I just expect to enjoy the moment and hopefully lot of awerness will spread thru youwecan today [sic]!'[26] He also thanked the doctor who treated him in the US, the BCCI and the National Cricket Academy for the support he got while he was going through the toughest phase of his life. And Yuvraj was showered with love and support from all directions.

Cancer is debilitating to sportspersons in more ways than one—not only is it difficult to cope with the disease, but it's also harder to keep their bodies in good shape, despite following a strict diet and exercise regime. And while Yuvraj focused on healing, the world kept moving on. So when he finally made a comeback and earned a place in the team all over again, many thought it was out of sympathy that he was selected, and many times, the incredible—and often excruciating—effort that he put into his practice sessions was overlooked. However, Yuvraj focused on his game and carried on, as he had always done.

Yuvi had been selected after a month and a half of gruelling practice. After the first match against New Zealand at the ICC World Twenty20, he played against Afghanistan in Colombo on 19 September, scoring 3/24. He ended up being the highest wicket taker for India in the tournament. His return to cricket post cancer was led by his performance with the ball, and that, too, in the T20 format. In the ten T20s he played from September to December 2012, he showcased his best statistics in bowling—he produced his career best of 3/17 against England at Wankhede, and took a total of 15 wickets in 2012, his highest in a year. He also won three MoM awards and one MoS award.

However, Yuvraj had a rather underwhelming 2013, where he averaged under 20 runs per innings in both the T20 and ODI formats. From 2014 to 2016, Yuvi was out of the ODI team but remained focused on T20 cricket. In fact, as far as IPL went, Yuvi was still in high demand. As mentioned earlier, in 2014, he was bought for ₹14 crore by RCB, and in 14 matches of that IPL season, he averaged 34 runs, with 3 fifties, and scored his career highest score of 83 in just 38 balls against Rajasthan Royals. He enthralled audiences with 7 sixes and 7 fours in that innings. Obviously, in the next (the eighth) season of IPL in 2015, Yuvi was in hot demand. He was bought by Delhi Daredevils for a massive ₹16 crore—a new record for the highest amount shelled out by an IPL team on a single player. But that season he managed to get only around 250 runs in a total of 14 matches and averaged only 19 runs per innings. In spite of this, knowing Yuvraj's reputation as the comeback king, in the next season of IPL, in 2016, he remained the Indian player with the highest price tag, bought by Sunrisers Hyderabad at ₹7 crore. Shane Watson had that year managed a bigger amount of ₹9.5 crore. In that season, he averaged a modest 26 runs per innings. After a great IPL season in 2014, Yuvi had a rather average 2015 and 2016.

In spite of a dry run, Yuvraj, who had now turned thirty-five, was still patiently working towards his comeback in the ODIs. And like always, he made it back. Playing in the Ranji Trophy for Punjab in October 2016, Yuvi amassed 672 runs in five games, which included his highest all-time score of 260 runs against Baroda and a fine knock of 177 against Madhya Pradesh. Yuvraj was now knocking on the doors of the ODI team. Meanwhile, the winds of change were blowing in the Indian team-selection meetings. In early January 2017, BCCI made some big announcements about the ODI series with England. Yuvraj was brought back into the ODI fold after a gap of three years; and Dhoni was replaced by Kohli as the captain of the ODI and T20 teams. A new era had begun and Yuvi was on the bus too.

About Yuvi's selection, the chief selector M.S.K. Prasad said, 'He has done extremely well in domestic cricket and [hence] given a due chance.'[27] Indeed, Yuvraj was, at that point, the highest scorer in that Ranji Trophy season. Though he missed the last leg of matches for his state Punjab (owing to his wedding), with 672 runs in five matches, he topped the list for his state.

When the series against England began, Yuvraj grabbed the opportunity with both hands. In the very second ODI in Cuttack in January 2017, he scored a stunning 150 and, in the third and final game in Kolkata, he scored a gritty 45. In that series, he hit a total of 210, at an average of 70 runs per innings.

The second ODI in Cuttack was indeed a special one. India was tottering at 25/3, but Yuvi and Dhoni added a record 256 runs for the fourth wicket to take the team total to over 380. Yuvraj slammed his career best of 150 off 127 balls, while Dhoni hammered 134 off 122 balls. The southpaw's match-winning knock had 21 boundaries and 2 sixes. His wife, actor and model Hazel Keech, was delighted, saying 'fierce' should be his middle name. Even though Yuvraj was restrained in his celebrations, it was evident he was a happy man when he got to the three-figure mark. It was his fourteenth ODI hundred and his first in almost six years. The last time he had reached the mark was against West Indies in Chennai during the 2011 World Cup, when he was in the best form of his life. And the greatest thing about his comeback was that he broke his previous highest ODI score of 139, which he had scored in 2004—a full thirteen years back. He was just twenty-two then! In the process, he overtook Tendulkar's record run tally in the ODIs against England, and accumulated 1,478 runs in 36 matches. And to add to it all, Yuvraj was declared the MoM. It felt like the good old times again.

Kohli was vociferous in his praise for Yuvraj after he hit 150. He said this was exactly what they had expected from the star. Yuvraj responded warmly by acknowledging that he would have retired, if not for Kohli's support. This was the third major comeback after his cancer treatment in 2012.

The final match against England in Kolkata was a dead rubber, but Kohli's boys were in no mood to get complacent while chasing 322. Once again, the openers fell, and Yuvraj had Kohli for company at the other end. The pitch started playing tricks under the lights, and Yuvraj even received a nasty blow on his chest from a bouncer by Jake Ball. But Yuvraj batted with caution and saw off the spells from Ball, Chris Woakes and Liam Plunkett, before launching into Ben Stokes for a couple of boundaries. The English bowlers kept testing Yuvraj with short balls, but to no avail. Yuvraj kept pulling and hooking the short balls for fours and took the pressure off Kohli. The duo added 65 runs for the third wicket, before the captain fell for 55. Yuvraj added another 31 runs with Dhoni, before getting out to a mistimed shot on 45, but by then he had already done his job.

Praising the Yuvraj-Dhoni partnership, Tendulkar said, 'Amazing partnership between superstar and rockstar.'[28] This kind of support from Tendulkar had always given Yuvraj the necessary push.

Learning Tip

Never give up, even when times are
bad. Keep working hard. Times will change.

'It feels great; it's been a while since I got a hundred. I came back after recovering from cancer. First two, three years were hard. I had to work hard on my fitness, I was in and out of the team. I was not able to get a permanent spot,' Yuvraj said, while addressing the media in the post-match press conference. 'Self-confidence is always there when you have the backing of the team and captain. I think Virat has showed a lot of trust in me and it was very important for me that people in the dressing room trust me...'[29] the 35-year-old star added.

Getting breaks is tough; making comebacks is tougher

The story of Yuvi's comebacks is both fascinating and inspiring. His 17-year career has seen unparalleled ups and downs, but for every trough in his career, Yuvraj has bounced right back to reclaim his spot on the Indian team and prove his worth as a lead contributor. Yuvraj's charismatic and confident demeanour has made his comebacks look easy, but each has been more hard-won than the other. After all, how many players who started their cricketing career around the time he did have managed to stay on for so long? Playing a sport at the highest level for a long duration is tougher than it looks. And for Yuvraj, it was far from easy. First, to maintain the highest standards of performance, his game had to be comparable to or even better than that of the dozens of younger players entering the sport every year. Someone or the other is always knocking on the selectors' door. But there is place only for fifteen in the team, so he needed to remain among the fifteen best cricketers in the country all the time. Secondly, during Yuvraj's career, there were fundamental changes in cricket formats—T20 was introduced and then IPL came in. With four forms of cricket being played, it could have been both tough and confusing to decide where to focus on. And since each format required a different pace, technique and mindset, adjusting to each format could get difficult. Thirdly, he had to overcome personal challenges such as maintaining form, and coping with injuries and family issues. And finally, there was the cancer.

In every profession, one faces similar challenges on the way to building a successful career. As one tries to achieve success at higher levels, the challenges get bigger. The journey from having many passions to choosing one, excelling in the field, performing at national and international levels and then staying there can be difficult.

So how does one successfully play a long innings in his chosen field? What did Yuvi do to keep making those comebacks and then excelling, again and again?

The key to making successful comebacks

The very first prerequisite to success is steely determination, and a never-say-die attitude to keep going after every fall. While this may sound easy, the real struggle is in practising it. Though determination has much to do with one's inherent nature, depth of passion and support system, one can hone it too. The second requirement for success is self-confidence. When we are in bad form or face a number of failures, it is easy to give in to that sinking feeling. The thought that 'I am not good enough any more' keeps resurfacing. Motivating yourself, having positive people around you, having a good guide, reminiscing your good performances and getting some measure of success (even if in a familiar or a less challenging environment) can help boost confidence. It is also important not to pay heed to negative people who try to pull you down. In January 2017, when Yuvraj made a fabulous comeback by hitting his career best of 150 runs off 127 balls, Yuvi said, 'Never giving up is my theory. I never gave up, I kept working hard and hopefully, with other ODIs, time will change.' And then he added, 'I don't think about who is reacting to what. And neither do I read the newspaper, nor do I watch television. I just try and focus on my game and I wanted to prove a point to myself that I am still good enough to play international cricket.'[30]

Learning Tip
Steely determination and self-confidence are the first two prerequisites for success.

The third aspect of making comebacks is working towards improving your performance. Ultimately, it is your performance that will matter. This means you need to stay fit, practise hard, improve your technique and attune yourself to the changes in the rules of the game. After being out of touch, when asked about his fitness regime, Yuvraj said, 'I was in pain initially. Your body becomes slow and heavy, and you feel that it's not going to react. But slowly and steadily, things change. It took me over two years to get my body back in shape. For fitness, I had to work extra hours and change my diet completely. Ageing makes things harder. But with more recovery on the body and more sleeping hours, I made huge changes in my lifestyle.' One should also be ready to reinvent oneself, if required. Often, after one has scaled the heights of success, one finds it difficult to get back to basic preparations. On two occasions, when Yuvraj was not at his best, he had no hesitation in going back to the Ranji level to get some match practice so he could get his form and confidence back. It's important to always keep one's ego out of the picture and be ready to go down to the lowest level again for the most basic preparations.

The final element for making a comeback is to earn the faith of selectors, captains or bosses. No matter how good and self-confident you are, it is the selectors or bosses who will finally offer you the opportunity for that crucial comeback, especially when they have so many other options to choose from. It is wise to maintain a positive communication with them.

Learning Tip

It's important to always keep one's ego out of the picture and be ready to go down to the lowest level again for the most basic preparations.

Yuvraj's comebacks show the efficacy of the above approach. It can be summed up very succinctly in 'play hard, perform better, win games—in case of failure, don't give up, start from scratch, build your way up...play hard, perform better...' What is required is an unflinching mind and strict discipline. In Yuvraj's case, he has been unstoppable. Retirement is far from his mind—and who knows, maybe he is gearing up to take on the 2019 World Cup and smash another bowler for 6 sixes in an over and take away the Player of the Tournament award.

Adding Value As a Multitasker: Focusing On Strengths

In 1983, when India was playing in the World Cup tournament in England, no one put even a penny on the Indian team. Before 1983, India had participated in two World Cups (1975 and 1979) and had managed to beat only one team. The Indian team itself didn't think it could win the cup, even though Captain Kapil Dev in his pep talk told his boys they could. All through the tournament, India kept putting in surprisingly brilliant performances and, finally, in a stunning and unbelievable victory, brought home the World Cup on 25 June. So what had worked in India's favour that year? It had four very good all-rounders in the team—Mohinder Amarnath, Madan Lal, Roger Binny and Dev. Amarnath contributed brilliantly in both the semi-final and the final, and was adjudged the MoM in both of these matches. In the semi-final against England, Amarnath took two wickets and gave just 27 runs in 12 overs, helping restrict England to 213 runs in 60 overs. When India batted, Amarnath scored 46 runs, which included 4 fours and 1 six. The final win, too, could be attributed largely to the all-rounders' performance. In a league match against Zimbabwe, when India was struggling, it was salvaged by Dev. India was going under at 9/4 as early as the sixth over, when Dev walked in. He stood strong at the crease even as he kept losing his batting partners—Sandip Patil, Binny, Ravi Shastri and Lal—at the other end. He stood the ground for 53 overs and scored 175 off just 138 deliveries, with 16 fours and 6 sixes, and remained unbeaten till the end. What a brilliant performance with the bat, when his primary role was of a bowler. In fact, playing with an average of 60 runs per match and a strike rate of 109, he hit a total of 303 runs in just eight matches. His unbeaten 175 against Zimbabwe was the highest score in that entire tournament. In the list of highest partnerships in the tournament too, Dev featured twice—once alongside Lal, hitting 62 together, and the other alongside Syed Kirmani, hitting 126, where both were at the crease till the end of the innings. If this was his prowess with the bat, with the ball he managed to get 12 wickets in eight matches. He had an economy rate of 2.9. His best performance was against Australia, when he took 5 wickets after conceding only 43 runs. But what is rarely spoken about is Dev's performance as a fielder. With seven catches in just eight matches, Dev was the player with the highest number of catches in the entire tournament.

Surely, India won the 1983 World Cup thanks to its all-rounders. Over the years, the cricketing world became more and more conscious of the role all-rounders played in the team. Sunil Gavaskar rightly predicted in the 1990s that the days of cricket to come would be an 'era of all-rounders'. Interestingly, before the 1992 World Cup, Gavaskar had predicted a win for Pakistan, perhaps spotting the strength of the all-rounders in the team then. Indeed, in the all-important final match against

England, it was the all-round performance of Akram that sealed Pakistan's victory. He scored 33 runs off just 18 balls and took 3 wickets, for which he was named the MoM.

It was becoming evident that a good all-rounder could be a team's winning card. Apart from scoring important runs, he could also get crucial wickets that could tip the scales in his team's favour. Jacques Kallis and Shaun Pollock of South Africa, Imran Khan and Shahid Afridi of Pakistan, Ian Botham and Andrew Flintoff of England, and Shane Watson of Australia are a few examples of great all-rounders.

If in 1983 India's all-rounders contributed to India's World Cup victory, in 2011, it was another all-rounder who carried the team on his shoulders to victory. And in this case, it was Yuvraj Singh.

Between 1983 and 2011, India did have great all-rounders such as Shastri and Irfan Pathan, but it has not been as fortunate as South Africa and Pakistan when it comes to all-rounders. Shastri was a hard-hitting middle-order batsman and a canny left-arm orthodox bowler. In the 150 ODIs he played for the country, he scored a total of 3,109 runs and grabbed 129 wickets. Much before Yuvraj, it was Shastri who hit 6 sixes, way back in 1985. It would be a good twenty-two years before the feat could be repeated by Yuvraj, in September 2007. Pathan, on the other hand, was capable of opening both batting and bowling performances for the Indian side. In just twenty-nine test matches, he had scored an overall 1,105 runs and taken 100 wickets. In his 120 ODI matches, he had scored 1,544 runs and grabbed 173 wickets. His hat-trick against Pakistan in a test match at Multan remains one of his most cherished moments on the field.

But in 2000 came Yuvraj, who redefined the idea of all-round performance. Earlier, cricket was all about each player specializing in a skill—so one would be either a batsman or a bowler. In which case, if one were a batsman and failed to perform on the crease, it would be unlikely that he got another chance to contribute to his team. This continues to be the fate of many teams even today.

But having an all-rounder increases the probability of the player contributing to the team in more than one way. That is why having all-rounders on the team is always a good idea. In recent times, India has often relied on Ashwin, Ravindra Jadeja and Hardik Pandya for all-round performances. In the 2017 test series against Sri Lanka, Kohli was asked what the team composition was like for the first test, and he said, 'We have three fast bowlers and two all-rounders in R. Ashwin and Ravindra Jadeja.'[31] This reflects how the selectors and the captain look at them. When most batsmen don't perform, there is a possibility that Ashwin or Jadeja, or both, will perform to save the batting order. Yuvraj's contribution to this shift in selectors' mindset with regard to all-rounders is paramount.

In the Indian team, the best all-round performances in recent times have come from Tendulkar, Ganguly and Yuvraj. Tendulkar, in his 1998 match against Australia, hit a 141 and also took four wickets, giving away just 38 runs. Ganguly, on the other hand, in a 1999 match against Sri Lanka, hit 130 and remained unbeaten at the crease, while also taking four wickets, giving away 21 runs. The third, Yuvraj, is remembered for his performance in the 2008 ODI series against England. In the first ODI, India won by a whopping 158 runs, thanks to Yuvraj's fantastic batting display of 138 off 78 balls, which included

6 sixes and 16 fours. Yuvraj was adjudged the MoM. For a star performer like him, if this was a good game, an even better performance awaited fans in the second ODI of the same series against England on 17 November at Indore. India had won the toss and chosen to bat first. The decision was turning out to look like a bad one. While Gambhir as the opener hit a 70 off 76 balls, Sehwag left the crease with just 1 run. Suresh Raina and Rohit Sharma didn't perform either and left the ground with just 4 and 3 runs each. But then came Yuvraj and smashed a 118 off 122 balls. He hit 2 sixes and 15 boundaries in that game, with a strike rate of 96.7. The other batsmen got very few runs on the scoreboard, and with great difficulty India managed to put up 293 as a target for the English side. England was waiting to avenge the humiliating defeat in the previous game. When they came out to bat, they lost an early wicket. Raina made Ian Bell go back to the pavilion on a splendid run-out, with just 1 run. Yuvraj, as though his performance with the bat wasn't enough, came around to bowl and got Matt Prior out, who had looked like he would settle down for a good score. From there, Yuvi went on to claim 3 more crucial wickets that could have won the game for England. Though Owais Shah had hit a 58 off 78 balls and begun to look undefeatable, Yuvraj got him out for a leg before. Petersen, the captain, was also sent back by Yuvraj by a stunning delivery. What was surprising that day was the energy he had, despite batting for almost half the innings. He bowled a full ten-over spell like a regular bowler, gave away just 28 runs and grabbed 4 key wickets. That day Yuvi scored 40 per cent of India's score and took 40 per cent of its total wickets. One simply doesn't know if this innings is to be cherished for his batting or for his bowling prowess—he

was brilliant at both. In the second ODI too, he was rightly given the MoM award. This performance launched him into the list of best all-rounders in India.

Yuvraj has had some really good all-round performances on several occasions. As early as 2002, when it had been just two years since Yuvraj had joined the team, his skills were evident during the NatWest series in England. In the second match, England had won the toss and elected to bat first. The Indian side managed to restrict them to 271. Bowling 7 overs, Yuvraj grabbed 3 wickets. Later, while batting, he hit 64 off 65 balls. India won the game with 6 wickets remaining. Here, too, Yuvraj's performance was rightly recognized. Despite Marcus Trescothick having hit an 86, and Sehwag and Dravid having scores above 70, Yuvraj was adjudged the MoM, thanks to his all-round performance.

In that NatWest series, India managed to get to the finals. There, too, Yuvraj's role was crucial to India's victory. England won the toss and elected to bat first. The Indian bowling side couldn't perform well and the Englishmen managed to hit 325 in 50 overs. India had to then chase this challenging target to win the game. Though Sehwag and Ganguly managed to put some runs on the board, Dinesh Mongia, Tendulkar and Dravid all left the crease early. Then came Yuvraj, who stayed on for a longer period and shared a noteworthy partnership with Kaif. Thanks to Yuvraj, Kaif got enough time to stabilize himself at the crease. In that final against England, Yuvraj stood by Kaif as he looked to threaten the English side. Their 121-run partnership helped India win the game—and the trophy. On several occasions, Yuvraj has contributed to important knocks of other batsmen on his team as well.

But his and Dhoni's partnership have a special place in fans' minds. When thinking about a favourite match, the 2011 World Cup comes to mind. In 2005, Dhoni and Yuvraj had scored 158 against Zimbabwe; they again scored 148 against Australia in 2009 to win the game. Dhoni and Yuvraj became the best finishers on the Indian side. If it was the two of them at the crease, Indians could be assured not only of victory, but of top-class entertainment too. Such partnerships have had a crucial role to play in making Yuvraj the reliable cricketer he is. Apart from excellent performances with bat and ball, he has been a huge support to his teammates as well. This is what makes his role truly multidimensional.

In the 2011 World Cup, Yuvraj set several memorable records as an all-rounder. In the game against Ireland in Bangalore, India won the toss and elected to field first. The Irish team had a good start, with William Porterfield, the captain, putting up a good 75 off 146 balls. Though Zaheer Khan had managed to take two crucial wickets by then, it was Yuvraj who got the captain out, which was necessary for a breakthrough on the Indian side. From then on, there was no stopping Yuvi. He went on to take 4 more wickets. He ended with a five-wicket haul and that, too, in a World Cup game. The Indians managed to stop the Irish team at 207. Thanks to a brilliant bowling spell—with Yuvraj taking 5 wickets and giving away just 31 runs in 10 overs—Ireland lost all wickets in 47.5 overs. Then, with the bat too, Yuvraj performed to ensure India's victory. He was the highest run scorer on the Indian side, with 50 off 75 balls, with three boundaries. India won the game and Yuvraj was again handed the MoM award. He was the first player in the history of the game to hit 50 runs and get 5 wickets in the same match in a World Cup. In that tournament, Yuvi became the first all-rounder in history to get more than 300 runs and 15 wickets in the same World Cup. That was when he proved that an important all-rounder can not only perform well, but do so at crucial stages in the game to ensure the team's victory.

In 300 ODIs, Yuvraj has taken more than 110 wickets. That is an average of at least 1 wicket in three games. In the T20s, in 58 games he has taken 28 wickets. That is an average of 1 wicket in every two games. Among cricket fans, batsmen usually enjoy a slightly exalted position, which puts the spotlight more on batting prowess rather than on bowling and fielding. As a result, Yuvraj's score and performance on the crease gets a lot more attention and praise than his achievements with the ball. For instance, his performance for Kings XI Punjab in 2009 was a treat for cricketing fans. On 1 May 2009, RCB was playing against the Kings. RCB won the toss and chose to bat first. Bangalore lost early wickets, but Robin Uthappa and Kallis came to RCB's rescue and gave it some stability. After trying out a few things on the field, Yuvraj was brought in to attack. Kallis began with an early boundary off Yuvraj. The next three balls also got some runs on the Bangalore side. But then Yuvraj's famous determination kicked in and he bowled the next one at full length, which Uthappa tried hitting over the mid-wicket but instead launched it high in the air, leading to a brilliant catch at the boundary by Simon Katich. In the next delivery, Kallis tried hitting the same shot that had got him an earlier boundary, but this time Yuvraj bowled the ball flatter and faster. It held its line and flicked the bails right off the off-stump. Yuvi had gotten 2 wickets in just 2 balls and was on a hat-trick run. But the next over was Piyush Chawla's and Yuvi had to wait his turn. When he got to bowling again, Yuvi brought in a slip to increase the pressure on Mark Boucher. Boucher tried to hit the ball on the leg side but missed—and it hit the stumps plumb. The umpire declared him out—Yuvraj had got his hat-trick! What thrilled the spectators even more was that, in the same match, he hit a half-century too. This one came fast, in just 33 balls. That day he was the centre of the game and again adjudged the MoM. But more amazing than perhaps the hat-trick itself is the fact that this was the same ground on which he had got his 6 sixes off Broad. The Durban stadium and the people of the city were indeed lucky.

Talking of hat-tricks, this wasn't the only time Yuvraj got one. In the same tournament, he got another against Deccan Chargers at Johannesburg. The Kings played first and set a target of 135 for the Chargers. Yuvraj had hit a 20 off 18 balls and, later, with the ball, performed even better—he got Herschelle Gibbs out for 26, Symonds for 25 and Venugopal Rao for a duck. He gave away just 13 runs in that game and managed an economy rate of 3.25. But unlike the last time he had got a hat-trick, this time his team won the match. In this match, too, he was given the MoM award.

Apart from these, Yuvraj has around six spells in which he took 3 wickets against formidable teams such as South Africa, England, Pakistan and New Zealand. Twelve times he has had spells where he took 2 wickets, again against teams such as Australia, New Zealand, Sri Lanka and Pakistan. It so happens that of all the batsmen sent off by Yuvraj, England's Pietersen has been the most dismissed. Many of us will remember how a hassled Pietersen made derogatory comments about Yuvraj's bowling, calling him a 'pie-chucker' and deriding his bowling as 'filth'. Yuvraj, who realized—gleefully—that he had managed to get to Pietersen, retorted the next day, 'I like that name.' Adding fuel to fire, he added, 'I got up in the morning and read the paper and wondered, "What does this [pie-chucker] mean?" So I asked a few people and they told me pie-chucker meant a useless kind of bowler. It shows KP hates getting out to me, and if a useless bowler is getting him out five times, then I would say that is quite useless batting.'[32] He had the press in splits as he held court, staying impishly tongue-in-cheek as he made the English captain the butt of quite a few jokes.

In fact, Yuvraj has had a special feud with England's players. Flintoff and Pietersen are among the batsmen whose wickets he has gotten the most number of times, and Broad himself has been immortalized alongside Yuvraj for the six sixes. A number of Pakistani players, too, have felt the heat both from Yuvraj's ball and bat.

But how did Yuvraj turn out to be a good bowler? After all, he started out as a batsman, and in his early days, he was written off by Bedi. From the way he has evolved as a bowler and the opinions of those around him, it is clear that it was his sheer passion and will to make his mark in the bowling department too that made him good at it. Reetinder Singh Sodhi, who played with Yuvraj in his younger days, said, 'He [Yuvi] wanted to be an all-rounder... [He] would try his hand at bowling, though there was nothing exceptional about him as far as bowling was concerned. He never bowled in the matches then at the junior-cricket level, but he would keep practising at the nets... He worked very hard on his fielding for over an hour after the nets.'[33]

So Yuvraj wasn't a born bowler—it was an acquired skill for

him, rather than a natural one. In fact, he started out as a left-arm medium-pacer but switched to spin after a back injury. Various selectors have watched his bowling skills closely and analysed his performance, and their views, too, suggest that he learnt the art of bowling the hard way—through hours of practice and a burning desire to be counted as a bowler of merit. Former Indian batsman Praveen Amre, who coached Raina and Uthappa, observed that Yuvraj's improvement as a bowler had a lot to do with the experience he gained as a player. He said, 'It looks like he isn't doing much, but he has learnt how to bowl to a field, and perhaps more importantly, he makes the batsmen play him. He gets a lot of caught and bowled chances and most of the times, he takes them. He draws on his experience as a batsman and bowls in areas that batsmen are generally uncomfortable in... A lot is made of how he takes the pace off the ball, but that is only part of the story. If you just take the pace off the ball, the batsmen will eventually get the better of you. But he keeps varying his pace and that makes the difference. These are subtle variations, and with every match you can see him grow as a bowler.'[34]

Former chairman of the selection committee of the BCCI, Kiran More, too, acknowledged that Yuvraj had gradually honed his bowling skills to emerge as an effective bowler. 'When I was chairman of selectors, he would not really concentrate on bowling. He would come in and just roll his arm over. But now he bowls a lot. The other day, I looked up his statistics for ODIs and found that he has over 100 wickets now... On the face of it, he seems to be pretty innocuous but his line and length is deceptively good. He doesn't get the ball to turn a lot—in fact, he even doesn't know which ball will turn. But then who said that you need the ball to turn square to take wickets? His dismissal of Ian Bell was a classic left-arm bowler's dismissal and even though he isn't a frontline bowler, you can count on him to bowl a good 15-20 overs in a match and that's important,'[35] he said.

Former Indian spinner Venkatapathy Raju, who was also a selector, decoded Yuvraj's method of trapping the batsman with his intelligent bowling. Raju said, 'See, he is a good bowler. He has good height—which gives him natural flight and a very clean and strong action. But I think his greatest advantage is that he is under no pressure when he comes in to bowl. No one expects him to take a wicket, and he always has his batting to fall back on. That allows him to experiment. He is dangerous because he is a clever cricketer. He uses his experience to find chinks in the batsman's armour.'[36]

In the fielding department too, Yuvraj was a class apart, especially in his younger days. All three captains he has played under—Ganguly, Dravid and Dhoni—would change every field setting but let Yuvraj stay at the point position. If it wasn't for the on-field brilliance of Yuvraj, many wickets taken by Indian fast bowlers (who often strayed wide of off-stump) would have been boundaries, and countless matches would have been lost. But if the ball was in the air and headed for point, everyone knew it would be clinched.

Knowing one's limitations: focusing only on strengths

Though being an all-rounder is a coveted position in the team, trying one's hand at too many things can dilute one's core strengths as well. Interestingly, while Yuvraj's career offers inspiration for becoming an all-rounder, it also offers lessons on how one should avoid chasing areas in which one is not that strong.

Yuvi always dreamt of performing well in tests, but his career statistics suggest that he didn't have as many great moments in test cricket as in the ODI and T20 formats. But then Yuvi wanted to perform well in all spheres of cricket. That is how he trained himself to be a good bowler too. And given his craving for excellence, he never gave up his dream of doing well in test cricket either.

Yuvraj made his ODI debut in 2000, but his test debut came in 2003 against New Zealand. He is one of the few players who have a lower batting average in tests than in ODIs (generally, test averages are better). But it's not like he does not have memorable test performances. He scored his maiden test century in less than a year, against Pakistan in Lahore during the second test of India's tour to Pakistan in 2004. Incidentally, all his three centuries in tests were against Pakistan and within a span of three years—from 2004 to 2007. In his early years, he did show promise in test cricket. In 2004, he impressed Captain Ganguly, who vouched for Yuvraj's place in the test team. In an interview in June that year, Ganguly categorically said that Yuvraj would be an opener in the tests. 'Yuvraj is a class act. A person of his stature and ability should not be kept out of the team. I think there is a slot for him as an opener. I am pretty much sure that with his ability and mindset, he will definitely get used to it,'[37] Ganguly told reporters in Bangalore, when asked about his plans to include Yuvraj on the test side.

In December 2008, Yuvi had a memorable innings with Tendulkar, when India was playing its first test against England in Chennai. In that match, Yuvraj scored 85 not out and put up an unbroken partnership of 163 with Tendulkar to defeat England. It was the fourth-highest successful run chase in history and the highest in India. This is regarded as one of his best test performances.

But to be truthful, he didn't have a sustained, record-breaking run in test cricket the way he did in other forms of the game. Yuvraj played only 40 test matches between 2000 and 2018 of a total 194 that India played. In fact, he did not play any test match after 2012, when he returned to cricket after his cancer treatment, though he did make some great comebacks in T20 and ODI. He was the lead contributor and won MoM and MoS awards in a record number of ODIs but, interestingly, was never an MoM or an MoS in any test match in his entire career.

It was often pointed out that Yuvi could not maintain consistency in his test career, and discussions on how he didn't fit into the test team began within two years of his test debut. The title of 'one-day cricketer' sat lightly on his shoulders. But we know that Yuvi is a fighter who doesn't give up. In an interview in March 2005, he said, 'That is my goal for this year. I want to do very well in the ODIs to build myself as a strong contender for the tests. Being labelled as a one-day player obviously doesn't help anyone. I have a test century against my name and I think that is enough proof that I belong in this league.' When asked about allegations that he tended to play in patches, he was honest in his reply. 'I think so, yes. I need to work on that. I bat well for four to five matches and then there is suddenly a lull in my performance. I definitely need to get more consistent,'[38] he said.

But things didn't change much the following years. In 2006, just a year after this interview, he acknowledged that there had been ups and downs for him in the tests, and that he would try to be more consistent.

But in 2007, the year in which he was part of only two out of ten test matches India played, things still hadn't got better. 'It's frustrating not to be able to play tests,'[39] he said. Three years later, in 2010, when he was again part of only three out of fourteen test matches India played, the situation remained the same. When an interviewer asked him how eager he was to return to the test squad, Yuvraj promptly said, 'Very eager! As I said, things haven't fallen in place for me in the last year and a half, and I just need to concentrate on whatever cricket I get to play, whether it is Twenty20 or ODIs. If I get selected in tests, it will be great.'[40]

The fact that he didn't play any test match after 2012 grated with Yuvraj. In 2015, he was asked, 'As a constant in Indian cricket's hierarchy in the past decade, you have made several transitions—for example, from junior to senior cricket—but which, according to you, has been the most difficult?' To this he said that rather than a transition, it was a particular time— when he struggled with test cricket—that he found the most difficult. 'I used to play one test and then be out of the team, and return to domestic cricket. So I used to play one series, then play domestic test cricket for four to five years before returning to the squad. This was my most difficult period.'[41] A year on, in 2016, he was again asked, 'With all the talent that you have, do you feel you could have done better in test cricket?' He responded, 'Yaar, when you've been the twelfth man of a team for seven years, and you have greats like Tendulkar,

Ganguly, Dravid, Sehwag and Laxman, it's difficult to get an opportunity...' But he was also quick to add what he could have done better. He said, 'There were times when [in tests] I couldn't convert my sixties and seventies into hundreds. So I think that's where I lacked. Instead of three, if I had six to seven hundreds, I'd have been happier, but it's not easy to score hundreds at No. 6.'[42]

Learning Tip

Be aware of your weaknesses,
but don't let them break you.

But Yuvraj still did not give up. The important thing here is that while he was aware of his weaknesses, he did not let them break him. He was confident about what he had achieved till then, and continued trying. In another interview the same year, in 2016, when he was asked what was the one new achievement he wished to accomplish at that point, Yuvraj replied, 'I think if I finish my career with 70-80 test matches, and play the 2019 World Cup, that will be a huge achievement. That's my target.'[43] The never-say-die attitude was still intact.

So, should Yuvi have been adamant about chasing his test-cricket dream till as late as 2016, especially when he wasn't a young lad any more, or should he just have focused on ODI and T20, where he had a far better track record? Probably the latter, at least after his return to cricket after cancer. After all, it is not uncommon for even the best players to focus on only a few forms of the game as their career progresses.

One thing to ponder when it comes to his IPL matches is

that there was a reason why he was sold at the highest price in not one, but two, IPL seasons, right after he came back from his cancer treatment. Even after he did not make it to the World Cup team in 2015—despite having won the Man of the Tournament award in 2011—he emerged as the most expensive player, at ₹16 crore, in the IPL 8 auction. There was a reason why he was the first Indian player to cross hundred sixes in T20 matches. The answer is that he was just more naturally suited to playing a hard-hitting and fast game, rather than playing defensive for the long days and sessions of test cricket.

Many famous personalities in cricket have thrived because they knew what their strengths and drawbacks were. Dhoni is a classic example. When he realized he was falling out of form and getting old, he dropped out of T20 and tests to focus on ODIs. In fact, he also gave up (or lost) his captaincy. Now that was the best captain India had seen giving up his captaincy; obviously, people were shocked to see him go back to being just another player in the team. But maybe Dhoni and the selectors thought this would be important for Dhoni himself and for the Indian team. Tendulkar is yet another example. He tried being the captain of the Indian side, but after failing to perform on several occasions, he relinquished the post. This helped him focus on his game better and do what he was good at—scoring runs and centuries.

Yuvraj, too, like Tendulkar, had chosen to give up his captaincy. The few attempts he made at captaincy showed that he couldn't take up the responsibility of so many things at the same time. In fact, in April 2013, Ganguly, one of India's most respected captains, revealed that the Pune Warriors management never thought of Yuvraj as 'captaincy material' after the debacle in the 2011 IPL season. Yuvi probably realized, too, that he could not be as good a captain as he was a performer and, unlike his test-cricket dream, decided not to pursue it. It was a smart decision, as it freed him up to focus on his own game.

There are important lessons here. Wanting to excel in all fields is an admirable trait—and a coveted one—but it is important to understand where one can't achieve beyond a point. As we saw, Yuvraj wasn't great at captaining teams and playing in test cricket. He gave up the aspiration of captaining a side—which benefited both him and his team—but when it came to test cricket, Yuvraj kept pushing. Despite trying to better his test game, he has only been partially successful. But he still believes he can make it big in test.

Lessons from Yuvi's career

If you have only one skill, it is inevitable that one day you will stagnate and become redundant. Excelling in a dynamic environment will require you to have multiple skills and the ability to acquire new skills and unlearn old ones that are no longer useful.

The corporate world today rewards people who can work multiple roles for the organization. In the world of business, one never knows what challenges will come up. It always works to the advantage of a company to have people who, apart from doing the job they are hired for, can quickly work to fix other things as well or learn new skills based on the company's evolving strategies. Having an all-rounder's mindset, thus, helps professionals to reskill, in case the business environment changes. They, thus, have an edge over the others when it comes to getting a job—and retaining it.

So how does one choose between being an all-rounder and just focusing on one thing? Well, there is no specific formula. Being an all-rounder gives one flexibility; specialization gives one depth. Being an all-rounder gives one protection from failing in one category and allows one to contribute more. On other hand, being a specialist gives one focus. However, it is also like putting all one's eggs in one basket.

So how do you decide? When you don't do well in one type of format, should you give up (because maybe that format is not for you) and focus on other formats, or keep fighting it out? That is one of the most difficult calls in any profession. Even for Yuvraj, switching between 20 and 50 overs proved difficult. When an interviewer asked him, 'Now that you play in three forms, is it harder to switch into improvising in Twenty20s or to building the big innings in tests?', Yuvraj said, 'Actually, after playing Twenty20 if I suddenly have to shift, I find it tougher to shift to one-day cricket than test cricket. Earlier, 50 overs would look like too few overs, and now, after Twenty20, 50 overs look like you have so much of time. It's a limited-overs format, but for me that is tougher to switch to than to test cricket. For me, switching from 20 to 50 overs, mentally you have to shift very quickly. The 50-over game plans require much more thinking than Twenty20, where you are going bang-bang. Test cricket is very different. It has changed and maybe at a faster pace, but a cricketer knows what is needed. Preparation is of a different kind. The ball changes. You want to leave a lot of balls outside the off-stump. You're trying to get set, you know that.'[44] It was this acknowledgement of the challenges he faced and the amount of work that he knew needed to go into his game that kept him afloat.

An all-rounder who pushes against his walls to ultimately demolish them but at the same time can tell the difference between a wall and a valley that cannot be crossed is a true inspiration to fellow human beings. Maybe Yuvraj was left out of tests because greats such as Dravid and Laxman occupied that space. Maybe he could have actually gotten better at tests if he didn't have to take the long break because of cancer. Or maybe he was only meant to be a great limited-overs player due to his aggressive style. Whichever was the case, the lesson for us is that we need to strike a balance between trying to be an all-rounder and focusing on becoming a specialist.

The risk of being jack of all trades, master of few

On the question of sticking to one strength versus diversifying, the trick is to be flexible enough to change your focus areas in response to your changing environment. But when you are doing well and the environment appears stable, it is better to not try out too many things. Also, building on one's area of strength helps one excel faster, rather than trying to overcome one's weaknesses. So if one is an excellent athlete but can act only moderately well, there is a better chance of achieving big success by chasing the field of sports rather than trying to become an actor, even if one is more inspired by film stars.

It is good to think of being useful to the team and doing more for it, but to achieve the highest peak of performance and be well known for something for years, one should focus exclusively on something and aspire for specialization. Doing too many things can get one temporary fame and satisfy one's urge to chase the many things one likes, but to be known for a long time for something, deep specialization is key. That is why even Dravid had resisted when he was being made to play the role of wicketkeeper in the team—he knew he would rather focus on batting.

Learning Tip

To achieve the highest peak of performance, focus exclusively on something and aspire for specialization.

With age, responsibilities increase, and it helps to limit one's focus on a few areas (unless you have a team to cover wider areas). Yuvraj talked about this in one of his interviews. 'My priority will always be cricket. I'm a married man now, so my wife is also a priority. And the brand is also a priority... Everything is a priority,' Yuvraj said. 'It is tough [managing the brand, cricket and personal life]. It is an ongoing process. You have to work extra hours. I think with maturity in life, you learn to balance all these things and at the moment I am able to do that,'[45] he added.

These are the words of a mature, seasoned player—and that's what one should aspire for. Because future generations remember those who are masters at something, rather than just jacks of all trades.

Commitment With Class

L ike in all other fields, in sports, too, there are those who
play the crucial role of keeping fans hooked to the game,
becoming, in a way, ambassadors of the sport. In football, one
remembers the Argentinean superstar Maradona and the way he
waded through his opponents on the field. His dribbling skills
on the field have been admired for ages now. Other footballers
have praised the 'Golden Boy', as he was popularly called. Michel
Platini, former French midfielder and president of the Union
of European Football Associations, said, 'Diego was capable of
things no one else could match. The things I could do with a
football, he could do with an orange.'[46] Even Lionel Messi, who
has come to be known as one of the greatest footballers of all
time—having won the Ballon d'Or five times, the European
Golden Shoe four times and numerous trophies for his teams—
holds Maradona in high regard. He one said, 'Even if I played
for a million years, I'd never come close to Maradona. Not that
I'd want to anyway. He's the greatest there's ever been.'[47] Pelé
has scored more goals, Messi has won more trophies; and both
have lived more stable lives and careers than Maradona, but it

is the latter who has achieved a status more iconic than any other in football. His style, his performance and his public aura have made him irreplaceable. So why do some sportspersons get such adulation from their fans, despite there being other players with better records? Well, it is not just because they are greatly skilled, but also because they possess a magical *style* and an alluring *elegance*. Apart from their mastery over the game, they have something undeniably attractive and pleasing about them.

Sportspersons who are widely followed have their own signature styles. Usain Bolt's famous 'to the skies' hand gesture, Dhoni's helicopter shot, Tiger Woods' fist pump and Rafael Nadal's trophy bite have all put a style stamp on their games. Ganguly is revered for his aggressive captaincy, Dravid is known for his calm steadiness when batting and Tendulkar is remembered for his perfect shot selection and execution at the crease. Thanks to their unique styles and appealing personalities, they have made a firm place in their fans' imagination, and continue to do so even after they have retired. Such sportspersons possess 'class'—a combination of style and elegance that one is usually born with and which cannot be acquired through practice.

In Yuvraj's case, too, many would say being 'classy' is the secret behind his huge following and presence on the field. His stylish demeanour has ensured he has a special place in his fans' hearts, despite the many ups and downs in his career. Many experts have marvelled at how effortlessly suave he looks just standing at the crease with his bat—determined, confident and stylish. He is both brutal and elegant at the same time, and that is a rare combination. Left-handed batsmen, such as Brian Lara, are generally thought to be more naturally elegant to look at, but what sets Yuvraj apart is that he possesses a deadly combination of elegance, power and agility. These qualities make this strong, 6'2" lad a treat to watch on the field. With his legs firmly planted on the ground, without having to do a lot of footwork at all, Yuvraj can send balls zooming out of the boundary for fours and sixes. In the history of international cricket, Yuvraj ranks eleventh in the list of batsmen with the most number of sixes to their name. And he has achieved this feat in just 304 matches. His total of 155 sixes gives him an average of one six in every two games. In fact, only five of the players above him on the list have more games to their name than him. If Yuvi had played as many matches as them, given his average, he would probably have shot up the list.

Yuvraj's sixes have been a delight to watch. Being excited that they add to the team's overall score is one thing, but being delighted to just watch them as a spectacle is another. Yuvraj's opponents, who are equally amazed at the ease with which he hits sixes, view them in the hope of being able to crack his secret code. So far, however, they have all failed. Even before the era of T20, Yuvraj was a hard hitter. It was his comfort with hard-hitting that got him the world's fastest half-century in the 2007 T20 World Cup against England. He had an impressive strike rate of 362 in that match, with a total of three fours and seven sixes. Only Gayle, the other left-handed batsman famous for his shots, has been able to match this.

When it comes to sixes and quick runs, Yuvraj has been a stunning cricketer. And again I come back to the six sixes he hit in Broad's over. It all started with sledging, a tactic used by many bowlers to disturb the frame of mind of the batsman at the crease, who may already be struggling to score runs. If the batsman gets incited and hits the ball out of sheer rage, he often runs the risk of being caught—and that's what the bowler banks on. England has tried this trick on Yuvraj many times. In the Group E match of the inaugural 2007 ICC World T20 at Durban, Yuvraj had hit England's all-rounder, Flintoff, for two boundaries, and there was an exchange between them—now popular in the media—that riled Yuvraj up. Unfortunately, it was Broad who was to bowl to him next. What happened in that over has affected Broad's image for the rest of his life. Interviewers ask him even today how that over affected him. Poor Broad has found different ways of tackling the question—sometimes angry, sometimes funny and sometimes indifferent—but has not succeeded in shaking off his dubious legacy. While many batsmen have responded to sledging with words, heated arguments and even physical brawls, Yuvraj has set an example on how to counter sledging in style.

After that short exchange with Flintoff, when Broad delivered his first ball to Yuvraj, it was hit for a fabulous six. The next two balls, too, went flying over the square leg fielder and the covers respectively. Broad started panicking and Flintoff just stood at the boundary line shaking his head in disbelief. But the best was yet to come. As it took a little time for the ball to be brought back to the ground, the English team had a small 'conference'. Commentator Ravi Shastri had rightly noted after the first six that the argument with Flintoff could have 'charged Yuvraj up a bit'. And, boy, was the English team about to bear the brunt of that! Broad's fourth ball was hit over backward point for yet another impressive six. The English captain Paul Collingwood ran up to Broad and tried giving him some suggestions, but it was of no use—the next ball, too, went for a six over the midwicket. The crowd was up on its feet, and so were the commentators. It was five in five, and everyone was acutely aware that there was a stunning new record on the horizon. The fielding positions were adjusted to stop Yuvraj from hitting another six, but it made no difference to him—the balls wouldn't be on the field but outside anyway. Like a predator that crouches before an attack, Yuvraj crouched slightly as Broad advanced for the last delivery. The wide mid-on fielder was cleared this time for the final fantastic six of the over. Yuvraj had not only responded to Flintoff's 'ridiculous shots' comment but also created history. At the end of the over, when he walked down the pitch, Yuvraj was smiling at Flintoff. He had joined Shastri, Sir Garry Sobers and Herschelle Gibbs as the only batsmen to have accomplished the feat. But Yuvraj was the first in T20 history to have achieved it.

But wait, there is more to this incident. What is not as frequently narrated along with this incident is what happened in the next over. Flintoff came back to bowl. Yuvraj had just hit the fastest half-century in the history of the game, in just 12 balls, and now, with Flintoff back, he had to pay him back a little more. And Yuvraj hit a six again—this time the third ball of the over. Flintoff, and the cricketing world, learnt that evening who not to mess with. This spectacular feat has become an indispensable part of Yuvraj's public image and defines his batting style, attitude and, more importantly, class. He wasn't one to get into ugly brawls and mar the image of the game, but, in the same vein as Tendulkar and Dravid, chose to respond only through the bat.

After the match, when asked about this *blitzkrieg*, he said, '[Flintoff's words] got me really worked up. I was really angry and I just wanted to hit every ball out of the ground, just give it back. Sometimes it's good for you. Sometimes it backfires. But on that day I think it backfired [on] them.'[48] What a cracker of a match and post-match that was! Wouldn't his fans happily pay millions to just relive those moments?

Another day he lifted his team out of impending loss to a spectacular win was in the 2014 IPL. RCB was playing against Delhi Daredevils; RCB won the toss and elected to bat first. But the first major batsmen got out with very few runs—Gayle, Kohli and De Villiers were all gone at 22, 10 and 33 runs respectively. It was then Yuvraj's turn to bat, and that innings, he hit an impressive 68 off just 42 balls, with a strike rate of 234—the best by any batsman that evening. But what was memorable was the utterly splendid way he scored those runs for the team. He hit a total of nine sixes that evening, getting 54 runs off sixes alone, close to 80 per cent of his score. RCB picked up a vital 16-run victory that evening over Delhi Daredevils. Pietersen, the Daredevils' captain and a good friend to Yuvraj, said at the presentation ceremony, 'That man [Yuvraj] over there batted like an absolute superstar. We got undone by a brilliant innings... It's always good to see the good guys doing well.'[49] Kohli, RCB's captain, was ecstatic. 'I am glad that Yuvraj Singh has stood up. A lot of people had written him off, which I think should never be done to any cricketer, because we never know when one can make a comeback,'[50] he said.

As other players also have observed, it is this deadly combination of scoring runs and doing it in style that has made Yuvraj a favourite with so many people across the world. It is a delight to watch him play, and even captains of opponent teams who have suffered humiliating defeats, thanks to him, have never denied that.

Yuvraj was asked in a 2007 interview about how he enjoyed the game, now that he was older and had become a senior player on the team: 'It's interesting sitting with you and you speaking about youngsters. On the field you're like a kid yourself, diving around and hitting sixes. But you've quietly grown up and become a senior player, haven't you?' Yuvraj's response was, 'When I was a kid I used to try and hit every ball out of the ground. After playing one-day cricket and test cricket, I never thought I'd get a chance to play like that again ever. Twenty20 has given me the opportunity of playing like a kid again. I can just feel free and go out there and hit. Once a year, Twenty20 must come around!'[51] That is how much Yuvraj likes hitting the ball hard and getting his sixes. His flowing drives, lofted slogs and hook shots are all delights that cricket fans—irrespective of nationality—will marvel at for years to come.

What sets classy players such as Yuvraj apart is that they seem to achieve miraculous shots rather effortlessly. They rarely seem under stress on the ground and achieve milestone after milestone wearing a smile on their faces. That is why it is so pleasing to watch Roger Federer play tennis, smashing records year after year. And that is also why, when Yuvi returned to T20 cricket after overcoming cancer, he received the highest bids. The franchises knew that Yuvi not only performed well and remained a lead contributor to the team, but did so with class and style—a true icon in cricket. And who wouldn't want that on their side?

Staying committed to the cause

So is it fair to say that players such as Yuvraj are charismatic achievers mostly because they are 'gifted' with style and natural strengths? In other words, is it largely their 'class' that gets them adulation and success? No, certainly not. Dig deeper and you will find extreme struggles, sacrifices and resolve. Yes, it is the class that is the most visible in matches and public appearances, but there is unbelievable hard work that goes into making an achiever—all away from the public gaze.

Class gives the performer an edge and a start, but to get to the top and stay there, players have to make that class work for them. Yuvraj had to make concerted efforts to ensure that he didn't end up being just a short-lived spark—a stylish, entertaining player that shone bright for a brief period and then vanished. So how does one make class work for him/her over a long career tenure? Let's see how Yuvraj did it.

Commitment to improving skills and staying fit

Reetinder Singh Sodhi said of Yuvraj, 'He was about fifteen when I first saw him bat and I was fascinated by his sheer power. He had a god-given gift of timing. And on top of all this, he could run like a madman. He is also a hard-working guy... And I think, deep down, he had a very strong feeling that he will play for the country.'[52] Sodhi saw early on not just the classy side of Yuvraj's batting but also his determination to do well, which ultimately led him to excel in both bowling and fielding, areas that he wasn't always the best at. In a 2005 interview, Yuvraj said, 'I wasn't a very good fielder, to start with. But I realized that if I wanted to play one-day cricket, I had to be an excellent fielder. That's when I worked hard on it. You feel good about the fact that people say you are one of the best fielders in the side and that it is rubbing off on the others as well. Fielding is a very crucial part of one-day cricket and you can make a big difference with it.'[53]

After Yuvraj worked on his fielding skills, many have praised him. He recalls how, once in 2010, 'Sachin tells me, "If you stand at point, the team will save 15-20 runs. You just need to watch your videos of the last couple of years." I watch my videos sometimes and I surprise myself. I'm thinking, "Is that me?" When I speak to Jonty Rhodes, he tells me, "It gives me goosebumps to see you fielding." A guy like Jonty Rhodes is telling me. So I think about it. But if I am not able to dive properly or move to the ball quickly, I will not stand at point.'[54] With age and injuries, when he saw a decline in his stamina and skill, he gave up his position at point—but continued to work on his fitness to regain it. In 2011, when asked if his body was strong enough and what his fitness regime was like, he said, 'For me, physical fitness is crucial, as I have to maintain my stamina to run on field. For that, I exercise at least for 30 minutes every day—it could be running or swimming or weight training [thrice a week]. I also am careful about what I eat on a daily basis.'[55]

After his cancer treatment, this line of questioning remained a constant in his interviews. People were always curious to know how Yuvraj was feeling, whether he would regain his earlier form or if cancer had taken a toll on his body. In 2012, his fans were delighted when he said, 'I'm starting to feel better, eating a lot of organic food. Doesn't taste good, but I have to eat it. I'm starting to walk more… Hopefully I'll come back fast.'[56] Year after year the same questions would be asked, some to rile him and some out of genuine concern. In 2013, he was again asked a similar question: 'There are no medical restrictions right now?' And Yuvraj replied, 'No, there aren't. The doctors in America told me to go ahead and train when I finished treatment... But I also pay attention to what I am eating. I eat organic food, ghar ka khana, ghar ka ghee and makhan most of the time. I also managed to lose around ten to fifteen kg, which I had gained when I started bingeing on food immediately after I was cured.'[57] Thus, commitment also means that one should be ready to let go of things they love. After coming back from treatment, Yuvi went to France for a few months for oxygen training, where he learnt about diets and how to reduce body weight. He concentrated on eating good carbs and more protein. He ate brown rice instead of normal rice and opted for gluten-free flour. And as expected, he was asked, 'As a Punjabi you must love your food, right? How difficult has it been to stick to this regime?' Yuvraj just laughed and said, 'Yes, we [Punjabis] love our food. But sometimes you have to sacrifice to get back to where you were. I still like to binge-eat here and there. [But] mostly I am on a good diet.'[58]

Learning Tip

Commitment also means that one should be
ready to let go of things they love.

By 2015, the most-talked-about aspect of Yuvraj's career was how many times he had made it to the team and how many times he had been dropped. He was asked if he had ever thought of quitting. Yuvraj answered, 'You have your moments in life where games are disappointing and they don't go your way, but as I said, what do you play cricket for? You play your cricket to enjoy.'[59] This frank admission of his love for cricket won many a heart that day.

Yuvraj has also emphasized that being born classy means that a lot of things can naturally go one's way, but that as the years pass, commitment, focus and practice become equally important. In 2016, a wiser Yuvraj Singh said, 'I always tell them [the younger players] to get the best out of themselves. Tell them to always keep speaking to their coach. Always tell them this time isn't going to come back. Today you're 23-24, tomorrow…you'll be 30 years old, and you'll be feeling, "I wish I'd done a bit more." That's how I feel—I lost three-four of the best years of my game. Couldn't do anything about it, since it was for health reasons… It's very important to enjoy the sport, because if you're not, it becomes a burden on you, it's tough. I felt when I was playing junior cricket, I really enjoyed it—but when it became a profession, there were times when there was so much pressure from critics, from media, I couldn't enjoy it. I've started to enjoy the game again, and I feel that that is the most important thing for a cricketer.'[60]

Learning Tip

Along with class, commitment,
focus and practice are also equally important.

So the point is that to perform consistently, one has to be committed to the profession, sometimes to the point of letting go of things one loves.

Being prepared for mid-career crisis

Working professionals talk about a mid-life crisis in their careers after the age of forty. But in sports, especially physical sports, the career itself is short-lived, usually ending before forty, so the mid-life crisis starts in the thirties. But what is this mid-life crisis in sports? First, a sport such as cricket evolves continuously and the comfort zone in which one may have started their career can change. For example, in the late 1990s, when it was just ODIs and test cricket, the game was relatively slow and fielding standards were still not that high. Hence, if a cricketer was technically great but naturally slow, and not very great at fielding, it was still acceptable. But as the game became faster after the mid-2000s, with field restriction rules and the arrival of T20 cricket, he would have found it difficult to cope. So the new crop of players, with a natural attacking style, would get preference over 'senior players'. To add to it, after the thirties, one's body is no longer the same agile machine it used to be and injuries tend to take a more serious toll. One can feel that one is losing out to the next generation and the evolving style of cricket. Fortunately, for Yuvraj, who always had a naturally attacking style, T20 came as a boon, but he couldn't escape the other challenges of a mid-life crisis—such as injuries and natural body fatigue. But then, Yuvi was smart enough to make adjustments to ensure his place and performance in the national team, even after facing injuries and returning from cancer.

No matter how good and classy a player is, mid-life does not spare anyone and brings with it internal and external changes that one needs to be prepared for and fight against. Other than working harder on staying fit, maintaining a diet and practising well, one needs to manage one's ego to rebound from a mid-life crisis. One needs to handle the fact that while one is becoming a 'senior player', one's place in the team is also at a higher risk. Also, as a senior player, one often needs to put ego aside and go back to the basics. In cricket, that means that when one is out of the national team for whatever reason, it helps to play, even in domestic cricket, with unknown players, to get the practice one needs to regain form. On the occasions that Yuvraj lost his spot on the team, he fought hard at the domestic level to regain his position. His coaches, fellow players and selectors noted this commitment to the game and offered him a spot back on the team. In 2015, Yuvi said, 'Yes, you want to play the game till you enjoy it, whether you are playing at the domestic or the international level. It is hard to motivate yourself to play domestic cricket, but you also have to realize that it is the only way back. That was my motivation [sic] key to do well at that level—having an eye on the prize.'[61] Yuvraj has stressed on the fact that there will always be a phase in a long international career when things won't go one's way. But one needs to maintain focus and work hard. 'When you play international cricket for thirteen-fourteen years, it is always tough to maintain one level. Especially with my body—I have worked really hard in the last two-three years since my recovery—it has been up and down.'

Learning Tip

As a senior in a profession, it is important to be able to put ego aside and be ready to go back to basics.

One can only wonder at how well he has performed in first-class cricket, for whenever he has lost his berth in the Indian squad, it has been his performance in first-class cricket that has assured him a place back in the squad again. He has played an overall 134 matches and has 8,866 runs at the first-class level. He has hit 26 centuries and 36 fifties, with an average of 45. His highest score is an impressive 260. This gives us a picture of how dedicated he was even at the domestic level, so he could regain his lost position in the Indian team.

Learning Tip

Even when things don't go your way,
maintain focus and work hard.

Staying away from distractions

One of the side-effects of being classy and having a huge fan base is the number of distractions they bring. Be it cricketers, badminton players or athletes, it is often said that early success, glamour and limelight can 'spoil' the performers; if their performance drops, as is sometimes sadly the case, criticism in the media gets louder. Even with Yuvraj, there was rampant criticism around 2010 that he was losing focus on cricket. Even Dev once said (around the same time) that Yuvi needed to regain his focus on cricket. The same year he acknowledged something not many cricketers would have: he said that if cricket had 50 per cent distractions ten years ago, today there were 100 per cent. And his words ring truer than ever today. Coming from different socio-economic backgrounds, cricketers from across India fight their way up to the Indian squad. But once there, the popularity they get and the contacts they make can be overwhelming. There is a huge risk of glamour luring them away from the game towards practices that could potentially ruin their careers.

Apart from the glamour is the kind of money that flows into one's pocket at this level. Indian cricketers are some of the most well-paid sportsmen in the world. So with this sudden jump in wealth and attention, it is easy to get lost. But Yuvraj has been careful to not let these distractions get to him. He has been in the headlines for being the costliest player in the 2015 IPL, and has even been asked whether this puts him under pressure, but he has been dismissive. 'Not really,' he said on the eve of the Delhi Daredevils' match against Sunrisers Hyderabad. 'I was sleeping when the auction was going on. And I didn't tell anybody to give me that money. Whatever money would have been given to me, I would have [still] played IPL.'[63]

One of the things that many successful people do to avoid distractions—as Yuvraj also does—is to read fewer newspapers, not watch TV and stay away from social media. That allows one to focus on what matters—practice, fitness and performance.

Avoiding unnecessary controversies

The other thing that can be distracting to 'classy' icons is controversies. The world was in awe of Tiger Woods and considered him in the same league as greats such as Pelé and Muhammad Ali. But just after Woods became the first billion-dollar sportsman, the slippery side to his personality, involving sex scandals, emerged. As one distasteful fact after another was revealed, his world—and his career—fell apart. His wife filed for divorce, he lost all his sponsors, he suffered from injuries and his performance in tournaments nosedived. An icon fell, his image tarnished permanently. His class and skill took him to great heights of celebrity, but his compromise on ethics and a controversial lifestyle, though hidden from the public eye for a long time, finally took him down.

In cricket too, many players have been guilty of such wrongdoings. Danish Kaneria, Mohammad Amir, Mohammad Asif, Salman Butt, Sreesanth, Jadeja and Azharuddin all made sensational news for their unethical practices.

Learning Tip

Stay away from distractions and focus on what matters—practice, fitness and performance.

It becomes the responsibility of the player to avoid this side of cricket, which has the power to threaten the sanctity of the game and destroy the career of the player. And in this aspect too, Yuvraj has been sensible. In 2010, he said that his body language while playing for the country was such that no bookie would dare to approach him for match-fixing. Yograj Singh, Yuvraj's father, had once said that if Yuvraj was ever involved in match-fixing, he would shoot his son himself. This is again another glimpse of the kind of training that had gone into making Yuvraj Singh the man he is.

Be it as a great sportsperson, as a business tycoon or as a political leader, when in a position of power, it is tempting, to say the least, to misuse one's position. Keeping these temptations at bay requires enormous mental strength and commitment to one's profession and ethics. Yuvraj has been more than aware of this and has himself spoken about these distractions on many occasions. In an interview with *Aap Ki Adalat* in 2010, he said there was about a 95 per cent chance of getting spoilt in cricket and that he, too, had made mistakes, but learnt from them. He stressed the importance of honesty and ethics in the game, so one could have peace of mind, which is crucial to a good game.[64] If Yuvraj's on-field performances showed us what a classy player he was, his actions away from the public eye illustrate how one can convert class into winning performances. Natural class is often god's gift, but it needs to be followed up with persistent efforts, if one is to achieve success.

Brand Yuvi: Balancing Career and Commerce With Compassion

'*Jab tak balla chalta hai, tab tak thaat hai*' (only till your bat swings will you have fame and money): Yuvraj famously said in an advertisement for an insurance company. This rings poignantly true. A star is surrounded by people only till he is successful; very few will stand by him when he is not in the glare of the spotlight. To make it through such times—when one questions everything one has achieved so far—and eventually regain form, one needs immense inner strength and the support of those who truly love him—fans, friends and relatives. And one needs compassion. Detection of the cancer must have been one such moment in Yuvraj's life. When he was diagnosed, it wasn't his training sessions, his fitness or his class that stood by him—it was the love and compassion of his true friends and family, and the support of millions of fans across the world that helped him overcome it. One should never fight one's battles alone—it is crucial to rely on those around you.

The first, and most steadfast, source of support all through

Yuvi's treatment was his mother, Shabnam Singh. It is the one thing that kept him going when his treatment was on in the US. Yuvi said, 'I had a good set of friends, and a strong core system with my mother, who was 24X7 taking care of me. I had the blessings of my Guruji to come out of that traumatic phase and the love of the whole nation.'[65]

Right from his early days in cricket, when he had to deal with his disciplinarian father, Shabnam was the one person who offered him the love and care he so badly needed; and she didn't leave her son's side even for a day during his treatment. Fans have come to respect her too, as news of her constant presence by Yuvraj's side became public.

In an interview in 2012, Shabnam admitted that that phase was more painful for her than she ever let on. She had to fight her son's cancer as much as he did. She said that the cooking, the cleaning and the caring for her son got physically exhausting, taking a serious toll on her mental health too. She used to go through the days 'like a zombie'. She realized that being emotional about Yuvraj's condition would only make it more difficult for him to fight the disease, so she had to be careful to never break down in front of him. She recalls the influence Lance Armstrong had on Yuvraj's life. She said he read voraciously in those days, and Armstrong's autobiography *It's Not About the Bike: My Journey Back to Life* was crucial in ensuring that he returned to cricket like a true warrior. Yuvraj, too, acknowledged how his mother kept him strong in those times. 'I think my mother is stronger than me, and she really kept me going. There were times when I would weep like a child, but she never shed a tear. She stayed strong and made me stronger.'[66]

Yuvraj has talked about how he realized in those days who

his real friends were. Many weren't there when he needed them the most; they were fair-weather friends who came just for the stardom. But as things changed, he realized there were actually just a handful of people he could fall back on for support. He needed them to tell him that he would be able to overcome the difficulties; he needed them to stand by him and remind him of the many tough fights he had put up in the past. Kumble and Tendulkar were two such friends, who even visited him in the US. They had played with him and knew what would work on him. Yuvraj was delighted by a surprise visit by Kumble and later took to Twitter to tell the world how he felt: 'It was so nice of jumbo to surprise me. Great motivation and a happy day spent with the legend.'[67]

Tendulkar's visit, too, moved him. His love and respect for Tendulkar is no secret—he had even dedicated his MOS award for the 2011 World Cup to him. Both of them posed for happy photographs on the visit and Yuvraj has mentioned on several occasions the affection that Tendulkar showed him during his cancer battle. In 2014, when they were again playing together at Lord's, Yuvraj touched Tendulkar's feet to uproarious applause from the crowd. That game, Yuvraj hit a 132 for Rest of the World, which took on MCC XI. Yuvraj also hit Tendulkar for a six over long on before mistiming another ball in the same over and getting out. Tendulkar was happy to see Yuvraj back in the game and patted him on his back as he was walking back towards the pavilion. This made a world of difference to Yuvraj, who had just come out of his struggle.

Harbhajan Singh, who is one of Yuvraj's closest friends, also stood by him like a rock throughout. Yuvraj now recollects how Bhajji, as he is called, would talk continuous nonsense just to cheer him up. Many newer players, such as Kohli, have also been quite close to him. In 2016, Kohli said, 'I am very close to him. He is like an elder brother to me. I have always been very fond of him. He plays the game with a lot of passion. He is a wonderful human being, not many know that.'[68]

Support also poured in over social media. Actor Amitabh Bachchan tweeted, 'Shocked to learn of Yuvraj Singh down with cancer...Yuvraj if you read this, know that we all pray for you...All shall and will be well.'[69] We can only imagine how inspiring this message would have been for Yuvraj. Dia Mirza, Ameesha Patel and Vijay Mallya also tweeted in his support and assured him that they were with him and that they would pray for his speedy recovery. Prime Minister Narendra Modi and former Chief Minister of Jammu & Kashmir, Omar Abdullah, also sent him their wishes.

But apart from the love and support of friends and well-wishers, he also needed the best doctors and experts to help him through, and Yuvraj has recognized all those who have helped him fight the toughest battle of his life—Jatin Chaudhary, physiotherapist and acupuncture specialist; Dr Nitesh Rohatgi, oncologist; Nitin Patel, physiotherapist; Dr Einhorn, who treated him in Indianapolis; and Nurse Jackie.

He had support flowing in from different corners of the world. Mails, messages, tweets and bouquets from fans, and those who even flew in from India to visit him, were all crucial to his healing. The way his fans followed even the smallest update on his treatment and celebrated even the smallest sign of recovery was truly remarkable. This kind of fan base even off the field is truly a boon. When he played well, they were jubilant, but even when he failed to perform, they stood by him, always believing he would do better the next time. When he was diagnosed, they didn't move on to the next cricketer waiting in line for stardom—they stuck with Yuvraj through his worst times. And that kind of devotion is indeed difficult to come by.

This spirit can be seen reflected in a poster held up by a fan when Yuvraj stepped into the field for the first time after recovering from cancer. This was the second T20 against New Zealand that India played at Chennai. The poster read: 'Goodbye Cancer, Welcome Sixer.' That apart, Yuvraj had 27 guests in the stadium that day who had come just to watch him return to the game. It was an emotional moment not just for him but for the entire cricketing world. What's remarkable is that his fans have grown in number after he returned to cricket, and it doesn't look like he will lose them anytime soon.

In bad times, it's always true friends and well-wishers who come to haul you out of dark days. Hence, it's important to not neglect them when you are doing well. One should build and nurture an emotional bond with them, and Yuvraj has shown his compassionate side even during his good times.

Learning Tip

Don't neglect friends and well-wishers
when you are doing well.

Yuvi: the compassionate hero

After Sunrisers Hyderabad won the IPL in 2016, Yuvraj, then thirty-five, dedicated the maiden title to his teammate, Ashish

Nehra, who had missed the latter half of the tournament due to a knee injury. It was Yuvraj alone who remembered Nehra that day. It may be a small gesture, but it speaks volumes about the kind of person Yuvraj is.

During the ICC Champions Trophy 2017, by when Yuvraj had played 300 matches in his career, he posted a tweet crediting Ganguly for his success. 'My favourite captain was Sourav Ganguly. I learnt a lot from him and my career flourished under him the most. He infused the feeling in us that we could win a series abroad,'[70] Yuvraj said in an interview. Ganguly had long retired as the captain and even as a player in the Indian team, but Yuvraj hadn't forgotten the role he had played in shaping his career.

Yuvraj has always used his celebrity status to do good, and it's not every day that one comes across someone who does. On Sunday, 4 June 2017, a much-awaited India-Pakistan match took place. Yuvraj played an explosive innings, scoring 53 off 32 balls, with eight fours and a sixer. Awarded the MoM, the champ later won everyone's heart with his tweet. He wrote, 'My innings on #CancerSurvivorDay is dedicated to all the heroes & survivors. Also my thoughts & Prayers to all impacted in #londonattack [sic].'[71] Stars are often so immersed in their own lives and careers that they hardly care about the plight of the world—the hundreds around them who need help and attention. But Yuvraj has always made it a point to acknowledge the troubles that others around him go through.

And this wasn't the first time Yuvraj was dedicating his award to a cause. In 2012, Yuvraj dedicated his MoM award to Nirbhaya, the victim of a vicious sexual assault in Delhi that year, even as she was battling for her life in hospital. Yuvraj knew that this dedication and the tweet in support of victims in London would have an immense positive effect on the situation on the ground.

In 2015, when the team's all-rounder Axar Patel was facing criticism from his captain and was asked to improve his batting, it was Yuvraj who helped him out. Patel recalled this in a fond memory: 'Yuvi paa had told me to build a positive atmosphere around myself. He said that there will [always] be critics.'[72] That day again demonstrated the empathy and perceptiveness with which Yuvraj dealt with his teammates, always giving advice that heals and not hurts.

His maturity shone through in 2015, when he was not made part of the World Cup team. He had had an unimpressive season and been in and out of the team. But when news broke that Yuvi had not been selected, an enraged Yograj took to the media to tear Dhoni, the captain, apart. The TRP-hungry media flocked in to catch Yograj's comments, such as, 'If M.S. Dhoni is having personal issues with my son, I won't do anything, God will do justice. Pray India wins World Cup under your captaincy but nothing can be more sad that you behaved this way.'[73] Dhoni's image in the public eye received a blow and there was nothing anyone could do to change it. But Yuvraj took to Twitter to clear things out: 'Like every parent my dad is also passionate and I am sure got carried away always enjoyed playing under Mahi n would do so in future [sic].'[74] He also tweeted that he would like to meet Dhoni and congratulate him on his new fatherhood. This instantly took care of the unnecessary controversy brewing. It was Yuvraj's love and respect for his fellow player and captain that led him to promptly clear up any misunderstanding that could affect Dhoni and his public image.

Yuvraj also realized that the Punjab state team had difficulties conversing in English. This wasn't a problem when they were playing for Punjab, but when they played at the national level or in the IPL, the team faced a challenge. And so, to ensure that the boys knew at least basic English, so that they could communicate with the other teams, he introduced 'English day.' On these days, usually Sundays, the boys of the Punjab team would have to talk only in English. This way, many juniors under Yuvraj learnt the language, and they have remained grateful to him for this initiative. This again shows how Yuvi was never just about himself and that he had genuine concern for his fellow players as well.

Commercial ventures (VC) with social ventures (NGO)

The period when Yuvraj was being treated for cancer was the first time he could even think of something other than cricket. This phase was the beginning of Yuvi's social and commercial pursuits.

This phase of his life made him realize that he wanted to give back to the society that had showered him with so much love and support. This led him to set up his NGO YouWeCan, which works towards raising more awareness about cancer and providing patients and survivors with better facilities. The idea took shape while he was still in hospital. He shared his experience with fans on social media, posting pictures and talking about the several physical changes he was going through. All this sent out one clear message: FIGHT.

Armstrong's Livestrong Foundation, and the personal message the cycling legend sent to Yuvraj, also inspired him to start YouWeCan. When you know that others are praying for you to come out of your troubles, you know that the fight is worth it. For Yuvraj, the toughest battle he faced, both on and off the field, was cancer, and he realized that he couldn't have won it alone, without the support of the people around him. It was then that he got down to work, aiming to extend much-needed help and support to cancer patients.

Today, YouWeCan focuses on every aspect of the battle with cancer, be it creating awareness about its symptoms and chemotherapy procedures or helping educate kids who are cancer survivors. 'All in all, we believe your hope and help from the near ones give you enough courage to face adversity in its face [sic],' the YouWeCan website says.

Yuvraj had always used his fame and wealth to uplift those who needed help, but after 2011, it became a matter of giving back to society. When he posted those pictures of him during treatment on social media, it instantly resonated with thousands of cancer patients and gave them a sense of connect with Yuvraj that infused them with fresh hope. What they felt from him was compassion and not pity, which they were used to from the general public. Being a cancer patient himself, he knew exactly what these patients went through and the kind of help they needed. Monetary need is just one aspect of it; love and support can keep their hopes alive and make then feel that with just a little more struggle, one can start afresh. This compassion and commitment to a cause is reflected in the very name of his NGO, YouWeCan: you and I will put up a fight against this cruel disease.

While skills can get one impressive records, it is humaneness that turns one into an icon. And Yuvraj, without doubt, has transformed from a celebrity to an icon today—not just because of his sixes, but for all the support he has extended, and continues to extend, to those in need.

Many cricketers tend to fizzle out after the age of thirty-five. Their careers near the end and they usually don't have a plan for the second half of their lives. But Yuvraj knew what he had to do. While working untiringly towards early detection of cancer for better treatment, YouWeCan also invested in start-ups through YWC Ventures. Its portfolio includes EazyDiner, Startup Buddy, Moovo, JetSetGo, EduKart and Creator's Gurukul, among others. There's also YWC Fashion, which has established itself as a leading sportswear brand in India over the past few years.

When asked about the nature of work YWC takes up, Yuvraj said that its main aim was to create cancer awareness among people and remove the stigma attached to the disease. He added that there were a lot of Indians who lacked the money necessary for early detection and treatment, and that was where YWC stepped in. He also said that he wanted child cancer survivors to be able to study and go to school. In keeping with this line of thought, he started the 'Together We Can' campaign on Desiredwings.com to gather funds to give scholarships to young students. Since parents lose a lot of money on their children's treatment, the latter's education suffers. It is here that Yuvraj wants to intervene and help them out. Restoring children's dreams and providing financial assistance to parents who have lost everything in their children's cancer treatment is YWC's vision.

One may think that for a celebrity such as Yuvraj, it is easy to raise money. That is not true. 'When I approach people for support, they expect me to sit with them and take photos with them. I don't mind doing that, but it seems as though that's not enough [for them to make a donation] either. Moreover, most corporate houses have their own CSR initiatives and they have no room for other causes. This attitude towards charity needs to change in our country,'[75] he once said in 2016. To combat this problem and to ensure a steady supply of funds to the foundation, Yuvi launched the YWC Fashion label, profits from which go to charity. In September 2016, he even organized a fashion show that had Zaheer Khan, Harbhajan Singh, Chris Gayle, Ashish Nehra, Virender Sehwag and Rohit Sharma join him on the ramp.

For Yuvraj, it is not just about investing in business, but investing in a business that helps people. There are millions of entrepreneurs in the world, but very few are actually interested in giving back to people, rather than taking something from them. The very nature of Yuvraj's start-ups reveals a lot about him. In 2017, YWC Ventures invested an undisclosed amount of money in Startup Buddy, a Gurugram-based company that serves early-stage businesses. Founded in 2015, Startup Buddy provides services to start-ups in India and abroad that range from incorporation, accounting and taxation to project advisory, legal and intellectual-property-related work. His investment was in a start-up that offered valuable advice to those new to business and trying to figure their way out. In 2015, YouWeCan Ventures Technology Ltd was established to support online start-ups, including e-commerce firms, to build brands and encourage entrepreneurship. It was reported that YouWeCan planned to invest ₹40-₹50 crore in online start-ups in healthcare, travel, hospitality, real estate and media in the next three to five years.

A very important component of Yuvraj's business ventures is

compassion. In fact, one of his early investments was in training young boys passionate about cricket. The Yuvraj Singh Centre of Excellence at Pathways International School was set up to give budding cricketers in the school the facilities they needed to expand their talent. The centre, which is open to both students and the general public, is the National Capital Region's first cricket academy to offer indoor facilities such as bowling alleys, a swimming pool and a gym. And the academy has turned out to be a blessing for budding cricketers.

Yuvraj is careful when it comes to business and, just like his game, doesn't play rash shots. Like in cricket, he has sought help from professionals to keep a close watch on the market. The investment company, YWC Ventures, which provides an initial seed fund of ₹10-₹25 lakh per investment transaction to young entrepreneurs, was, at a point, run by a six-member team, which included chartered accountants, technology experts and management consultants.

All of Yuvraj's ventures have a uniquely human touch, which make them stand out in a world where it's all about the money. But for him, it is important to ensure that the country gains, even if a little, through his investments. Here is a list of start-ups he has been associated with in the past. Today this list is even longer.

- ▶ Beauty and wellness app Vyomo was a natural choice, as fitness has always played an important role in Yuvraj's life.
- ▶ Moovo, a technology-based booking platform for mini-trucks, also has a personal connect, as a large number of India's truckers hail from Yuvi's home state, Punjab.

▶ Bengaluru-based Cartisan, which helps customers book maintenance services for cars.

▶ Healthians, an aggregator platform of diagnostic labs and health-check-up facilitators.

▶ Edukart, one of India's top ten ed-tech start-ups.

▶ JetSetGo, a platform for booking private jets and helicopters. It is noteworthy that JetSetGo founder Kanika Tekriwal is also a cancer survivor.

▶ Fast food chain Carl's Jr.

▶ Black White Orange, which promotes celebrities and provides other branding consultancy services.

▶ Sports365, an online sports store, which also has the backing of Indian tennis star Mahesh Bhupathi.

▶ SportyBeans, a platform for teaching pre-schoolers ball sports in multiple locations. Kids can sign up for classes in cricket, baseball, tennis, golf, soccer, volleyball, basketball, hockey and rugby. This venture, which aims to foster a healthy lifestyle and team spirit among children, is probably the closest to Yuvraj's heart.

Yuvi the brand

Yuvi's life and career have inspired youth and grown-ups alike. So much so, that Yuvi has become synonymous with a fighting spirit, a never-say-die attitude, class, charisma, commitment and compassion. In his own words, 'The USP of my brand is "Live to Inspire"; it is the story of my life. Live, dare, inspire a lot of people [despite] whatever adversities they have gone through. So, it [is] an inspirational brand. The brand talks about my life journey.'[76]

The power of this USP has also been harnessed by a number of brands at various points in Yuvraj's career. He was signed by Microsoft as brand ambassador when the Xbox 360 video game console was launched in the Indian market in 2006. In 2007, Donear Suitings & Shirtings also signed him on as brand ambassador. Its executive director explained why Yuvraj was a natural choice. 'Yuvraj Singh is an all-rounder, a youth icon and has a great fan following. He represents dynamism, trust and durability, all of which symbolize our company. Looking at the all-round persona of Yuvraj and the brand attributes of Donear, we feel Yuvraj is the perfect representative for Donear.'[77] The tagline used by Donear—'If you can dream it, you can do it'—also seems perfect for Yuvraj.

In 2009, Birla Sun Life Insurance appointed Yuvraj, Sehwag, Raina and Sharma as the company's brand ambassadors and launched its first campaign with them for its 'Wealth With Protection Solutions' category. In 2013, Investors Clinic signed Yuvraj on as its brand ambassador. Explaining why, CEO Honey Katiyal said, 'We're extremely excited to have Yuvraj on board as the brand ambassador for Investors Clinic. He has a keen fighting spirit, which gels well with our efforts to strengthen our brand, while we relentlessly work towards maintaining our competitive edge.'[78] But Yuvraj has been part of several endorsements before, too; brands such as Reebok, Pepsi, Parachute, Hero Honda, Birla Sun Life and Royal Stag have all benefited from Yuvraj's image.

One brand that stood by Yuvraj during his lean period was Revital. Brijesh Kapil, Vice President, Ranbaxy Global Consumer Healthcare, said the company launched an aggressive marketing campaign immediately after the 2011 World Cup on a 360-degree platform focusing on TV, print, outdoor, online and digital space.

'After a tough phase, he has suddenly become a star performer and the man of the World Cup. Since we have been with him during his tough phase without caring what people said, we think this is the time to give everybody a fitting response, just like Yuvraj has done with his performance.'[79] Kapil said. Yuvraj's image in the public eye has been intrinsically linked to his various comebacks. But just like his game, he has ensured that the products also get a boost back into the market.

Yuvi today is a brand and an icon not only because he is a classy player, a fighter and an achiever, but also because he understands the importance of compassion in one's personal and public life. He has achieved that perfect balance of career, commerce and compassion. YouWeCan has worked wonders in the life of cancer patients, who now have the will to rise phoenix-like from the ashes to get back to life. YWC Ventures, too, helps small-time entrepreneurs with the edge they need to be important players in the competitive market.

One can see how Yuvraj's personal life has not been too different from his endorsements, his brand, his NGO and his entrepreneurship. It is this alignment between his personal and public life that has given his commerce a human touch, infusing it with a love and compassion that is rare in today's world. Here, too, Yuvraj stands tall among so many other celebrities by combining commerce and compassion. Can you think of a better hero?

Endnotes

1. https://www.hindustantimes.com/cricket/yuvraj-singh-wants-to-inspire-young-people-with-his-story/story-eiH88hfSxaeO6YcmtG7NTL.html

2. https://economictimes.indiatimes.com/small-biz/startups/yuvraj-singh-starts-new-innings-as-businessman-with-youwecan-ventures/articleshow/46831328.cms

3. https://www.indiatimes.com/sports/guess-which-actor-yuvraj-singh-wants-to-star-in-his-biopic-none-other-than-the-khiladi-himself-akshay-kumar-266832.html

4. https://timesofindia.indiatimes.com/sports/off-the-field/US-firm-to-produce-documentary-on-Yuvraj-Singh/articleshow/51175671.cms

5. http://www.openthemagazine.com/article/sports/the-making-of-a-champion

6. https://www.sportskeeda.com/cricket/yuvraj-singh-inspiring-story-cricket-cancer

7. https://www.indiatimes.com/lifestyle/self/yuvraj-singh-in-aap-ki-adalat-part-1-315404.html

8. https://www.hindustantimes.com/icc-champions-trophy-2017/yuvraj-singh-s-debut-in-icc-champions-

trophy-was-special-sachin-tendulkar/story-ynpynBgF2UT0LmoANDooLK.html

9. https://www.hindustantimes.com/india/plenty-at-stake-for-yuvraj-as-delhi-daredevils-take-on-chennai-super-kings-in-ipl/story-cXCQ79hJ43rM8XYlOt0f1K.html

10. https://www.news18.com/cricketnext/news/beating-the-four-time-champions-special-572717.html

11. https://www.news18.com/cricketnext/news/pietersen-doffs-his-hat-at-majestic-yuvraj-552591.html

12. https://www.cricketcountry.com/news/yuvraj-singh-talks-about-his-2011-world-cup-experience-200427

13. https://www.youtube.com/watch?v=u1jsrCjOPV4

14. http://www.espncricinfo.com/ci/content/story/315303.html

15. http://www.espncricinfo.com/story/_/id/22661621/yuvraj-singh-ruled-mirpur-test-ligament-injury

16. https://www.dnaindia.com/sports/report-2010-has-been-my-worst-year-yuvraj-singh-1483028

17. https://www.livemint.com/Leisure/QZWQsi11FWbnzOup7QxjdN/The-reeducation-of-Yuvraj-Singh.html

18. https://timesofindia.indiatimes.com/sports/new-zealand-in-india-2016/interviews/Happy-to-be-back-to-form-after-injury-Yuvraj/articleshow/6685738.cms

19. https://www.sportskeeda.com/cricket/yuvraj-singh-inspiring-story-cricket-cancer

20. https://twitter.com/yuvstrong12/status/167729030567698432

21. https://sports.ndtv.com/cricket/yuvraj-singh-posts-hair-gone-picture-on-twitter-1559382

22. http://www.espncricinfo.com/india-v-new-zealand-2012/content/story/581818.html

23. Ibid.

24. https://sports.ndtv.com/india-vs-new-zealand/today-is-my-biggest-day-since-world-cup-final-yuvraj-singh-1548236

25. https://twitter.com/yuvstrong12/status/244336591181578240?lang=enl

26. https://www.deccanherald.com/content/277324/yuvi-says-comeback-match-his.html

27. https://www.deccanchronicle.com/sports/cricket/060117/yuvraj-singh-given-a-new-chance-makes-a-comeback-to-team-india.html

28. https://www.indiatoday.in/sports/cricket/story/yuvraj-singh-mahendra-singh-dhoni-shah-rukh-khan-cuttack-odi-india-vs-england-955928-2017-01-19

29. https://timesofindia.indiatimes.com/sports/cricket/england-in-india-2016/virats-trust-was-important-as-i-could-have-retired-yuvraj/articleshow/56681500.cms

30. https://www.financialexpress.com/sports/never-giving-up-is-my-theory-yuvraj-singh/514942/

31. https://www.firstpost.com/firstcricket/sports-news/india-vs-sri-lanka-ravichandran-ashwins-selection-as-a-no-6-all-rounder-shows-teams-shift-in-mindset-4222009.html

32. https://www.mirror.co.uk/sport/cricket/yuvraj-singh-if-im-a-pie-chucker-kevin-367407

33. https://www.outlookindia.com/magazine/story/the-young-turks/216658

34. https://www.firstpost.com/sports/what-makes-yuvraj-such-a-dangerous-bowler-511627.html

35. https://www.firstpost.com/sports/what-makes-yuvraj-

such-a-dangerous-bowler-511627.html

36. Ibid.

37. http://www.rediff.com/cricket/2004/jun/13gang.htm

38. http://www.rediff.com/cricket/2005/mar/31yuvraj.htm

39. http://www.espncricinfo.com/ci/content/story/315303.html

40. https://www.dnaindia.com/sports/report-2010-has-been-my-worst-year-yuvraj-singh-1483028

41. https://www.sportskeeda.com/cricket/interview-with-yuvraj-singh-selection

42. https://timesofindia.indiatimes.com/interviews/Would-love-to-play-Tests-again-Yuvraj-Singh/articleshow/51936894.cms

43. https://www.sportskeeda.com/cricket/yuvraj-singh-hopes-play-2019-world-cup

44. http://www.espncricinfo.com/magazine/content/story/478169.html

45. https://www.crictracker.com/everything-is-priority-at-the-moment-yuvraj-singh/

46. https://www.goal.com/en-tz/news/7561/hall-of-fame/2014/11/12/6071731/the-flawed-genius-who-defined-a-generation-diego-maradona-is-one-

47. https://www.fifa.com/live-scores/news/y=2010/m=10/news=maradona-others-see-him-1326223.html

48. http://zeenews.india.com/sports/cricket/andrew-flintoff-tells-yuvraj-singh-i-will-cut-your-throat-off-read-yuvis-reply_1880391.html

49. https://sports.ndtv.com/cricket/live-blog-ipl-7-dd-vs-rcb-match-38-1518558

50. https://sports.ndtv.com/cricket/virat-kohli-slams-critics-

who-wrote-yuvraj-singh-off-1518524

51. http://www.espncricinfo.com/ci/content/story/315303.html

52. https://www.outlookindia.com/magazine/pwa_story_first/216658

53. http://www.rediff.com/cricket/2005/mar/31yuvraj.htm

54. http://www.espncricinfo.com/magazine/content/story/478169.html

55. https://completewellbeing.com/article/yuvraj-singh-i-have-a-strong-mind/

56. https://timesofindia.indiatimes.com/news/Yuvraj-Singh-meets-Pune-Warriors-team-mates-in-IPL-match/articleshow/12883626.cms

57. https://www.hindustantimes.com/brunch/yuvraj-singh-s-comeback-after-cancer-and-his-book-the-test-of-my-life/story-ugYvLMKdSiqBtK2haESdMM.html

58. https://www.firstpost.com/sports/interview-yuvraj-singh-on-his-fitness-regime-diet-and-the-motivation-to-comeback-2556936.html

59. https://indianexpress.com/article/sports/cricket/i-just-want-to-play-and-enjoy-my-cricket-says-yuvraj-singh/

60. https://www.news18.com/cricketnext/news/i-hope-to-play-until-2019-world-cup-says-yuvraj-singh-1290371.html

61. http://www.bcci.tv/australia-v-india-2016/news/2015/features-and-interviews/12357/want-to-win-matches-for-india-again-yuvraj-singh

62. Ibid.

63. https://www.firstpost.com/firstcricket/sleeping-auction-didnt-tell-anybody-give-rs-16-crore-yuvraj-2202218.html

64. https://www.youtube.com/watch?v=u1jsrCjOPV4

65. https://www.hindustantimes.com/cricket/yuvraj-singh-celebrates-life-and-a-glorious-cricket-comeback-on-world-cancer-day/story-gwrHfyiGSnKMevaavA5NXN.html

66. https://www.indiatoday.in/magazine/supplement/story/20120521-shabnam-singh-yuvraj-singh-cricket-world-cup-cancer-758359-2012-05-10

67. https://www.cricbuzz.com/cricket-news/50064/jumbo-surprise-for-yuvi

68. https://www.sportskeeda.com/cricket/virat-kohli-talks-candid-about-achievements-yuvraj

69. https://www.news18.com/news/india/amitabh-bachchan-shocked-to-hear-about-yuvraj-singh-444100.html

70. https://indianexpress.com/article/sports/cricket/my-career-flourished-under-sourav-gangulys-captaincy-yuvraj-singh-4706884/

71. https://twitter.com/yuvstrong12/status/871448015722213376?lang=en

72. http://zeenews.india.com/sports/cricket/how-yuvraj-singh-helped-axar-patel-deal-with-criticism_1838321.html

73. https://indianexpress.com/article/sports/cricket-world-cup/2294693/ms-dhoni-told-selectors-that-yuvraj-singh-was-not-needed-in-world-cup-squad-claims-father-yograj-son-differs/

74. Ibid.

75. https://www.hindustantimes.com/brunch/hazel-accepted-my-friend-request-after-three-months-yuvraj-singh/story-DG9EninDoXfKDUGeij23kO.html

76. https://yourstory.com/2017/08/ywc-fashion-yuvraj-singh-fit-healthy/

77. http://www.afaqs.com/news/story/19187_Donear-aims-a-sixer-signs-on-Yuvraj-Singh-as-brand-ambassador

78. https://www.business-standard.com/article/press-
releases/investors-clinic-signs-yuvraj-singh-as-brand-
ambassador-110120700118_1.html

79. https://www.business-standard.com/article/management/
brand-yuvraj-the-game-has-just-begun-111040600065_1.html